How NC

Doctor Cabot's

Copyrigh

Published by SCB International Inc. - United States

www.sandracabot.com
www.liverdoctor.com

ISBN: 978-0-9829336-6-4

HEALTH & FITNESS / Women's Health

Women's Health; Premenstrual Tension; Premenstrual Syndrome; Hormonal Imbalances; Menstrual Distress; Thyroid Problems; Progesterone; Natural Progesterone; Bioidentical Hormones; PMS; PMT; Infertility; Endometriosis, PCOS; Polycystic Ovarian Syndrome; Teenage hormone problems

Disclaimer

Notice of Rights

Dedication

This book is dedicated to women of all ages who have suffered, and continue to suffer needlessly, with hormonal imbalances. Natural progesterone is able to liberate us, so why is it one of medicine's best kept secrets?

This book will show you how to overcome premenstrual syndrome and the myriad of other hormonal problems induced by progesterone deficiency.

Women of all ages will shout *"Thank goodness for this eye opening book!"*

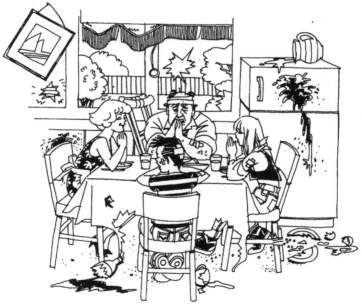

...and we are especially thankful that mummy's period is over for another month

Contents

About the Author

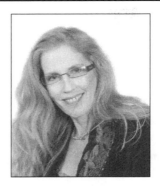

Sandra Cabot MD

Dr. Cabot is the Medical and Executive Director of the Australian National Health Advisory Service. She graduated with honours in Medicine and Surgery from the University of Adelaide in South Australia in 1975.

Dr. Cabot began her medical career in 1980 as a GP Obstetrician-Gynecologist and practised in Sydney Australia. During the mid 1980s she spent 6 months working as a volunteer doctor at the Leyman hospital, which was the largest missionary hospital in Northern India.

Sandra is the author of the Award winning *Liver Cleansing Diet* – the best selling non-fiction book of the 1990's and is still a best seller!

Dr. Cabot has also written many other ground breaking books which can be seen at www.sandracabot.com.

Dr. Cabot is an experienced commercial pilot and flies herself to seminars throughout Australia, often visiting remote areas. Dr. Cabot and her Beechcraft Baron aircraft do regular work for the Angel Flight Charity, which provides free transport for patients with severe disabilities in remote Australian areas. Dr. Cabot's aircraft has done several hundred flights since January 2007 for the Angel Flight Charity.

Dr. Cabot has conducted health seminars all over the world and has frequently lectured for health organizations such as The American Liver Foundation and the Annual Hepatitis Symposium. Doctor Cabot still has an active medical practice and does research into liver diseases.

Dr. Cabot believes that the most important health issues for people today are –

- The control of obesity and the prevention of diabetes
- Educating our children about self esteem, good diet and healthy lifestyle
- Making hormone replacement therapy safe and as natural as possible
- The use of specific nutritional supplements to treat and prevent diseases
- Educating doctors and naturopaths so that they can work together using evidence based holistic medicine to achieve the best outcomes for patients
- The effective treatment of mental and emotional illness
- A supportive and well educated community where people have the confidence and knowledge to find the best healthcare

Her free magazine can also be read on line at www.liverdoctor.com

Introduction

Balancing your hormones can save your marriage, as well as your husband's life. Maybe you don't care? Chances are that you are angry, frustrated, tired and just over it. That's your perspective and it's real and probably justified – hell who wants to be a perfect superwoman and mum and wife at the same time. The expectations on women these days, to be everything to everybody whilst under the influence of hormonal upheaval, can be enough to see you reach breaking point.

But over the years, I have seen plenty of marriages saved and some husbands have a lucky escape from an angry wife and thus I know the power and stress of hormone dysfunction. I have been truly impressed by the ability of natural progesterone to restore hormonal and mental equanimity to women within a short time of just a few weeks.

If you are a woman you may buy this book to help yourself or your daughters or perhaps to save your marriage. Your unsuspecting husband would probably not buy it, because he would think it's only a funny humorous book written in a sarcastic way. Well if only he knew just how much danger he was in, I think this book would appear quickly on the best seller list of the New York Times!

Hormones are beyond a doubt the most powerful chemicals in your body. They have the power to be physically and emotionally shattering or they can make you feel wonderfully alive. No one wants to live on a series of extreme highs or lows and we don't have to do that anymore because it's now possible to fine tune your hormones to avoid this *hormonal seesaw*. To feel really well most of the time, you need to achieve a balance in your hormones and this book teaches you how to do that. Many women feel confused and somewhat helpless and, as victims of their hormones, are desperately searching for ways to escape the prison of hormonal chaos.

Why are hormonal imbalances more common these days?

We are seeing a higher incidence of hormonal imbalances such as –

- Precocious puberty
- Polycystic Ovarian Syndrome
- Unexplained infertility
- Endometriosis
- Irregular menstrual cycles
- Premenstrual syndrome
- Premature ovarian decline
- Syndrome X – the chemical imbalance of insulin resistance which leads to excess weight gain

These hormonal disorders reduce the quality of women's lives and need to be addressed at a deeper level, where we are not just treating the symptoms of these problems.

The incidence of hormonal disorders in women has increased over the last 20 years, because of sociological, environmental and dietary factors, which include -

- Women have fewer children and have children later in life, which leads to a relative deficiency of the hormone progesterone.
- The chemicals we are exposed to in this toxic day and age. Most of these chemicals were developed during and subsequent to the industrial boom after World War II. These chemicals are capable of disrupting the function of the endocrine glands and are known as *endocrine disruptors*. They are able to attach to hormone receptors on the cell membranes and can block the action of our own naturally produced hormones. These chemicals include pesticides, plastics, polychlorinated biphenyls (PCBs) and solvents. They pollute the air, waterways and food chain and are found in many household products. We willingly and sometimes unwittingly ingest artificial chemicals such as MSG and aspartame in diet sodas and diet foods. These are known as excito-toxins because they over stimulate the nervous system causing disruptions in the hypothalamus and pancreas. This disrupts the endocrine glands and increases the risk of obesity. See www.dorway.com

- Dietary imbalances – we consume too much carbohydrate from refined flour products and sugar, which increases our insulin levels; this is called Syndrome X and causes weight gain and ovarian dysfunction. We consume too much unhealthy fat from hydrogenated vegetable oils and deep fried food. It is healthier to avoid the fatty parts of meat, as these often accumulate fat soluble toxic chemicals, so trim off the fat and remove the skin from poultry (unless it's organic). Deep fried foods are unhealthy because the fat becomes oxidized producing free radicals, which can damage the liver and endocrine glands. Hormonal imbalances can be greatly improved by food combining and detoxification of the body – for more information see www.liverdoctor.com and the book titled *The Liver Cleansing Diet*.

In this book we will look at how hormones affect your mental and emotional state, your nerves, the menstrual cycle, headaches and your energy.

This is a *save your life book* and gives you the tools to communicate effectively with your own doctor and to work with your doctor to gain control of your hormones. With the increased self understanding that you will acquire from this book you will have the confidence to be assertive with your healthcare providers to demand the type and quality of care that you need. Balancing your hormones naturally will free you to realize your full potential and enjoy good health. With the right information, you need not let your hormones ruin your life.

I work with a team of doctors and naturopaths in Sydney and Phoenix. You may phone my Women's Health Advisory Service for more information – in the USA phone 623 334 3232 and in Sydney 02 4655 8855 – and also visit us online where you can subscribe to our free e-newsletters and contact our helpful naturopaths to whom you can email your questions to ehelp@liverdoctor.com

If you would like an in-depth telephone consultation with a naturopath you can make a booking by calling +61 2 4655 8855. Information about our clinics is available at www.sandracabot.com

Dr. Sandra Cabot

1. What is a Hormone?

Hormones are body chemicals that carry messages from one part of the body to another. They are manufactured in specialized glands (endocrine glands) located in various places in our body and are circulated in the bloodstream to body cells where their presence makes a dramatic impact. *See Image 1.*

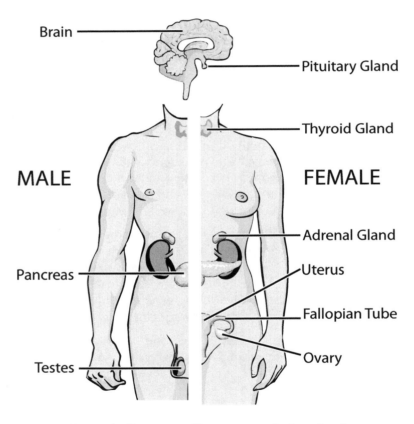

Image 1 - Diagram of hormone producing glands

Some examples of the many glands required to keep our cells functioning in harmony are:

- The thyroid gland, which manufactures thyroid hormone
- The adrenal glands, which manufacture adrenalin, cortisol, DHEA and other steroid hormones
- The ovaries, which produce the sex hormones estrogen, testosterone and progesterone
- The pituitary gland which manufactures hormones that control other glands

Compared to many other body chemicals, hormones are relatively slow acting in producing their effects upon our cells. Hormones determine the rate at which our cells burn up food substances and release energy and thus control the metabolic rate – this is of great importance to those who battle with a weight problem! Hormones also determine what metabolic products our cells will produce such as milk, hair, secretions or enzymes.

Hormones are extremely potent molecules and in some cases, less than a millionth of a gram is enough to trigger their effects. They are far too small to be seen even under a microscope but are easily and accurately measured with a blood test. After they have completed their tasks, hormones are broken down by the cells themselves or are carried to the liver for breakdown. Once broken down by the liver, hormones are then excreted from the body via the bile or urine or are used again to manufacture new hormone molecules. It is important to have a healthy liver in order to be able to achieve hormonal balance and your diet has a big effect upon your liver.

Hormones can be likened to chemical keys that turn and open receptors *(metabolic locks)* on the surface of our cells. The opening of these receptors stimulates activity within the cells of our brain, intestines, muscles, genital organs and skin. Indeed all our cells are influenced to some degree by these amazing hormonal keys. *See Image 2*

Without hormonal keys, the metabolic locks on our cells remain closed and the full potential of our cells is not realized. This could be compared to a corporation where the employees are unable to communicate with the managing director and are left to do their own thing. Such a corporation would lack any unified direction; this would result in chaotic dysfunction. This is precisely what happens in our cells without the correct type and balance of hormones.

Before hormone attaches to cell receptor (metabolic lock)

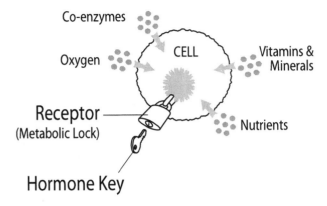

Co-enzymes

Oxygen

CELL

Vitamins & Minerals

Receptor
(Metabolic Lock)

Nutrients

Hormone Key

After hormone attaches to cell receptor (metabolic lock)

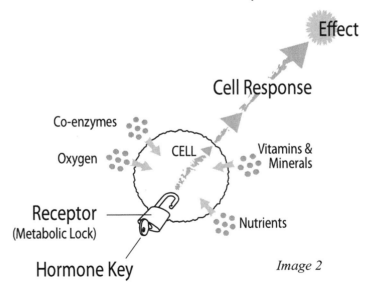

Effect

Cell Response

Co-enzymes

Oxygen

CELL

Vitamins & Minerals

Receptor
(Metabolic Lock)

Nutrients

Hormone Key

Image 2

2. The Premenstrual Syndrome

Katrina had married at the age of 19 against the advice of parents and friends. By the age of 22, she had two beautiful toddlers and a successful husband, who doted on his children. Katrina should have been blissfully happy, but she wasn't. For two weeks before her periods, she became morose, irritable and hurtful to her family. She lost interest in sex and felt ugly and unloved.

When her menstrual flow began, the dark clouds dissolved and she became her carefree self again but with bitter memories of how she had hurt those she loved. She became the caring mother and wife and resumed her painting and pottery, as an expression of her creative spirit. Life was good again until ovulation began and then, with monotonous regularity, the dark storm clouds gathered around.

Bettina, aged 37 had a vastly different lifestyle to Katrina. She was the typical career woman, an executive in a multi-national corporation. She told her friends that she had simply forgotten to have children and marriage was not on her agenda in the context of her sixty-five hour working week. There were many who envied her but underneath her cool executive veneer, Bettina was starting to crack. She jumped down the throats of her colleagues, mixed up appointments and became confused for about seven days before each period. She made obvious and serious mistakes and blamed others for not covering up for her inadequacies. The only way Bettina could cope during the week before her period was by drinking more alcohol and chain-smoking. She was wracked by intense headaches for three days before every period and needed frequent doses of painkillers to keep going. As soon as her period began, her headaches vanished and she became once again the cool, calm, collected executive with the seemingly perfect veneer. Deep down, Bettina knew that if this monthly imbalance continued, she would burn out by the age of 45.

Perhaps you can see yourself in these two very different women. As a doctor, I see hundreds of such cases in my surgery every year. It is the classic, woeful tale of Premenstrual Syndrome or PMS; it can also be called Premenstrual Tension or PMT. Most women will have heard of PMS or PMT, as it has received extensive coverage in the press and media, but it still remains a very misunderstood and poorly treated issue.

PMS and PMT is surprisingly common and surprisingly variable. About 50% of women in their reproductive years will notice unpleasant mental and physical changes in themselves sometime during the two weeks before the menstrual bleeding begins.

PMS is the medical term used to describe the collection of different mental and physical problems that may occur during the second half of the menstrual cycle. There are many different possible symptoms and the important clue is not their nature but the cyclical timing of the symptoms. If the symptoms are due to PMS, they will begin in the second half of the monthly menstrual cycle, sometime after ovulation, and will disappear once the menstrual flow begins. The symptoms will then reappear after ovulation occurs in the next menstrual cycle and so the cyclical repetitive nature of PMS will become apparent. *See Image 3*

Some women will notice symptoms for the full two weeks preceding bleeding, while others will feel unwell for only several days before bleeding. Some months may be worse than others with a variation in the intensity and type of symptoms.

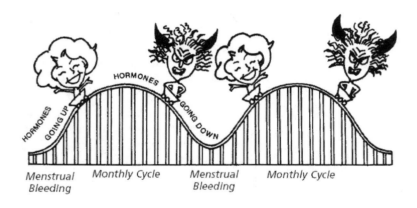

Image 3 - The Hormone Rollercoaster

There are many possible symptoms of PMS and indeed Dr. Katharina Dalton, a world authority on this subject, has identified 150 of them. Once again, it is not the type of symptoms but the cyclical relationship of the symptoms before menstrual bleeding that distinguishes PMS from other medical disorders. (Ref 3)

Common Symptoms of the Premenstrual Syndrome

Mental and Psychological Symptoms

Mental and emotional symptoms can include:

Depression, anxiety, irritability, sudden mood changes, aggression, hostility, alcoholic bouts, drug abuse, panic attacks, insomnia, fatigue, sleepiness, confusion, low self-esteem, paranoia, reduced concentration, exhaustion, reduced libido. Aggravation of manic depression or obsessive compulsive disorder may occur premenstrually and be relieved by the onset of the menstrual blood flow. Some of the more curious symptoms include creative urges or feeling *spaced out*.

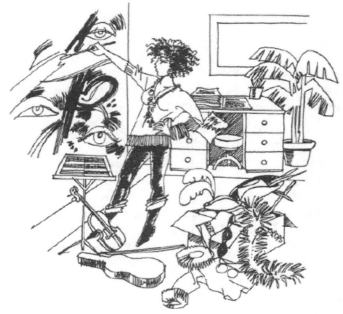

Some of the more curious symptoms of the PMS include creative urges...

Image 4

Physical Symptoms

Physical symptoms can include:

Headaches, including migraines, breast swelling and tenderness, fluid retention, abdominal bloating, low blood sugar, food cravings, sugar binges, dramatic changes in weight, clumsiness, poor co-ordination, fainting, acne, general aches and pains, backaches, muscle tension and spasm, spotting of blood, constipation and pelvic pain.

Another curious phenomenon is that of *premenstrual magnification.* This means that medical problems, such as allergies, mouth ulcers, genital herpes, candida, asthma, epilepsy, schizophrenia, arthritis and migraine, etc, may become worse during the two premenstrual weeks. During this time, there seems to be a reduction in general resistance and immune function. If you have an Achilles' heel, it is most likely to affect you in the Premenstrual zone.

What causes the Premenstrual Syndrome?

I well remember one evening in the country town of Grafton, NSW, relating Hippocrates theory on the causation of female hormonal imbalances to an entirely male audience. These men had come to listen to my after dinner talk about *How to be a perfect husband.* My mother had got me into this rather sticky situation, as she had delighted in 'setting me up' when the male dominated Lions Club had requested my services as an after dinner speaker.

During my talk, as I explained that Hippocrates had blamed a *wandering uterus* that travelled up to the brain and disturbed the emotions, a little man at the front of the audience became wide eyed and intrigued. I further related that Hippocrates' treatment for PMS was to entice the wayward uterus back into its rightful position in the pelvis by burning aromatic incense at the vaginal opening. At this juncture, the same man's jaw fell open and he looked relieved. After my light hearted dissertation, he came up to me and whispered in my ear saying that *"he had problems at home and did I have any of that incense for sale!"* It is amazing what desperate husbands will do!

After the Hippocrates treatment, it took until 1931 for doctors to realize that hormones had something to do with PMS! A certain Dr. Franks preached the theory that too much estrogen caused PMS. His treatment was even more drastic than that of Hippocrates, as he recommended large doses of laxatives to flush the demon hormones out of the body. Dr. Franks claimed great success with this treatment, which is little wonder, as the intense discomfort of the resulting diarrhea, was enough to drown out all the other woes of the PMS victim. Some women even had their ovaries subjected to radiation and consequent destruction in a desperate attempt to end their PMS.

There is no doubt that the monthly cyclical fluctuations in the levels of the sex hormones estrogen and progesterone play a large role in causing PMS. This is supported by the observation that PMS begins only after puberty, recurs on a monthly basis and disappears during pregnancy and after the menopause.

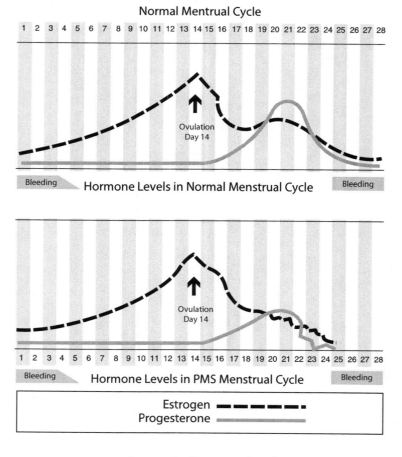

Image 5 - Hormone Levels

In PMS sufferers, it is after ovulation that the fireworks begin. In a woman without PMS, the levels of estrogen and progesterone remain in sufficient and balanced amounts between ovulation and menstrual bleeding. In a woman with PMS, the levels of estrogen and progesterone are out of balance with insufficient estrogen and/or progesterone between ovulation and bleeding. *Image 5*

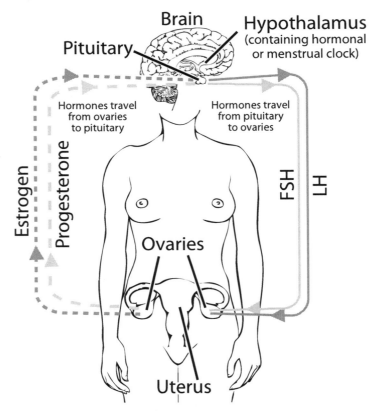

Image 6 - Hormonal Control of the Menstrual Cycle

Some researchers believe that it is the ratio of estrogen to progesterone that is more important than the absolute amounts of these hormones. They have found that women, who have too much estrogen compared to progesterone (estrogen dominance), have anxiety and tension. Women with too little estrogen compared to progesterone often complain of depression during the premenstrual phase.

Indeed, there are many subtle variations in the levels of sex hormones produced from the ovaries and a whole range of imbalances in all three ovarian sex hormones, estrogen, progesterone and testosterone can be involved. This accounts for the variation in PMS symptoms between different women and between different cycles in the same woman.

The study of the female sex hormones is called gynecological endocrinology and it is a relatively new medical specialty with still much to explore. We stand at the frontier of an explosion in the scientific discovery of how imbalances in sex hormones influence our mind and bodies. PMS is truly a Pandora's Box and we have now dared to lift the lid so that one by one, the hormonal demons will be tamed and controlled.

If you glance at *Image 6*, you will see the mushroom-shaped pituitary gland situated at the base of the brain. The pituitary gland controls and *speaks* to the ovaries by sending chemical messengers called Follicle Stimulating Hormone (FSH) and Luteinizing Hormones (LH) via the bloodstream to the ovaries. FSH and LH stimulate the ovaries to manufacture both estrogen and progesterone.

Ovulation occurs when an ovary releases a mature egg and the cells left behind in the ovary then form a small yellow colored gland called the corpus luteum. For the 2 weeks after ovulation, the corpus luteum manufactures the hormone progesterone, and if it is healthy, it manufactures sufficient amounts of this wonderful health promoting hormone *Image 7 and 8*.

How can you find out if you are ovulating regularly?

Blood Progesterone

After ovulation, the ovary normally produces the female hormone progesterone and your doctor can easily measure this in the blood around the twenty-first day of your menstrual cycle. If the doctor finds no progesterone in the blood, this will confirm a lack of ovulation. See *Image 8* which shows a normal ovulation cycle with plentiful production of progesterone.

Basal (resting) body temperature

Another way of determining when you ovulate is by measuring your temperature when your body is at rest. This method is cumbersome and not entirely accurate, but it can be used as a backup, in combination with other methods. This method is more useful for women who have regular menstrual cycles that are close to 28 days long. You will need to measure your body temperature with a mercury thermometer first thing in the morning when you wake up, before getting out of bed. Your body temperature remains fairly constant each day under normal circumstances, however just after ovulation your temperature rises by 0.3 to 0.5 degrees

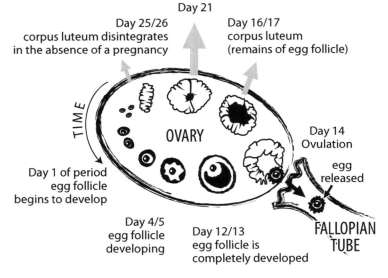

The grey arrows represent by their size the amount of progesterone produced

Image 7 - Monthly Ovary Cycle

Celsius, and remains elevated until your next period. The rise in body temperature is caused by the progesterone made by the corpus luteum after ovulation. Conversely, with a lack of ovulation, no progesterone is produced. Thus the post-ovulatory increase in basal body temperature does not occur.

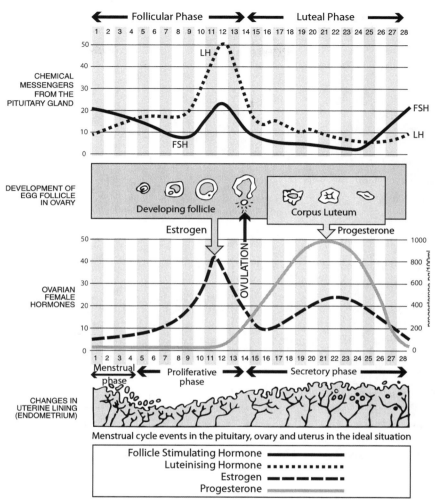

Image 8 - Menstrual cycle events in the pituitary, ovary and uterus in the ideal situation

A temperature chart must be measured over three cycles to obtain an accurate idea of your ovulation time. *See Image 9*

Note: Women are most fertile the few days before their basal temperature rises, and are least fertile when their temperature has remained elevated more than three days.

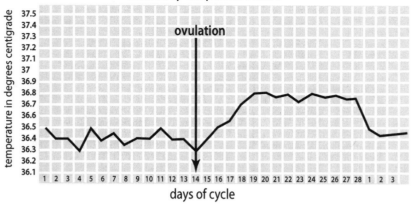

Image 9

Instructions for measuring your basal body temperature.

Use a mercury thermometer, as they are more reliable than digital thermometers for measuring small changes in temperature. Take your temperature the same time each morning, as soon as you wake up, by placing the thermometer in your mouth. You should only take your temperature if you have had at least 4 hours of solid sleep before waking. So if you have had a restless night, or gone for a bathroom trip four hours before waking, this method will not be as reliable. That may exclude a lot of women! For accuracy, your temperature should be taken at the same time each morning. Sleeping in late on the weekend can make it more difficult to see a pattern and link temperature changes to ovulation.

Several things can affect your temperature, thus making this method inaccurate; these include an infection or other illness, stress, alcohol consumption the previous day, allergies, iron deficiency, adrenal gland exhaustion, thyroid disorders and some medication. If used on its own, the basal body temperature method of tracking ovulation is not always reliable.

If you notice a rise in your basal body temperature after ovulation, and your temperature has remained elevated for more than 20 days, this could indicate you are pregnant.

Ovulation testing kits

There are several ovulation testing kits available in pharmacies that are very helpful for determining when you ovulate. Most kits work by measuring luteinizing hormone (LH) levels in your urine. Immediately before ovulation, the pituitary gland produces large amounts of LH, which triggers the release of a ripe egg from the ovary. Ovulation test kits detect a surge of LH in the urine, which indicates that ovulation will likely occur in the next 24 to 48 hours. This is your most fertile time and the optimum time for sexual intercourse that can lead to pregnancy. Ovulation testing kits are less reliable in women with short or long cycles, or women with polycystic ovarian syndrome.

Cervical mucus

Just before ovulation, there is an increase in the amount of cervical mucus which appears in the vagina, and this mucus is clear and slippery.

On the day of ovulation, there is a peak or maximum amount of this clear slippery cervical mucus. After ovulation the mucus becomes thick and opaque under the influence of progesterone.

Symptoms of ovulation pain

Many women who ovulate notice a short lived sharp pain on one side of the lower abdomen which is due to the egg bursting through the ovarian capsule at ovulation. It may be associated with a small amount of blood loss from the vagina and an increase in libido, and some women find it a very reliable sign of ovulation.

3. Does Nutrition play a role in PMS?

Nutritional imbalances and deficiencies can greatly worsen PMS. I have observed that many women obtain complete relief from PMS after improving their diet and taking nutritional supplements. You may, as I did originally, find it surprising that such simple and safe nutritional strategies can completely overcome the sometimes dramatic and severe symptoms of hormonal imbalance and yet, it is a demonstrated fact that I have seen countless times.

Can nutritional supplements help overcome PMS?

A number of studies have found that vitamin B6 in a daily dosage of 25mg to 100mg can give satisfactory relief of many PMS symptoms such as premenstrual headaches, fluid retention, irritability and depression in around 60% to 80% of women.

Vitamin B6 helps to regulate the brain's biochemistry and is necessary for the conversion of tryptophan to the brain hormone, serotonin.

Serotonin is a natural regulator of mood, sex drive, sleep and appetite. In my experience, vitamin B6 is much more effective if it is taken along with other B vitamins, such as vitamin B1 (thiamine), vitamin B2 (riboflavine), vitamin B3 (niacinamide), and vitamin B 5 (pantothenic acid). B complex vitamin tablets contain all of the B vitamins.

I had the pleasure of discussing women's health with the remarkable doctor, Lady Cilento, shortly before her death and she told me that she had had great success in alleviating PMS in thousands of women with one injection every four weeks of vitamin B12 (cyanocobalamin). This certainly has merit in women with poor diets, heavy menstrual bleeding or in those who are strict vegetarians or suffer with digestive complaints.

The antioxidant, Vitamin E, can also be most helpful because it is involved in the production of various hormones from the adrenal and pituitary glands, as well as the vitally important male hormones. Vitamin E is a superb antioxidant protecting the fatty membranes of our cells thereby improving ovarian function and reducing inflammation. Several studies have found it successful in relieving premenstrual breast pain and lumpiness.

Zinc and Selenium

Zinc and selenium play a vital role in human metabolism and have been found to be commonly deficient in the diets of western women in the reproductive age group. Zinc and selenium are necessary for proper function of the ovaries, and a healthy immune system and they promote healthy skin and hair. They could be considered minerals to enhance physical beauty. Many PMS sufferers should take a regular supplement containing these minerals. A common sign of zinc deficiency is white marks on the nails.

Selenium is able to reduce the symptoms of fibrocystic breast disease and has proven cancer preventative properties.

Magnesium

This mineral is often deficient in women, who consume a diet that is high in refined carbohydrates and sugar. Such a diet will deplete the body of the minerals chromium, zinc and magnesium. Women with PMS have been found to have lower levels of magnesium in their red blood cells, compared to PMS-free women. (Ref 8). Women with a magnesium deficiency often crave sugar and in particular, chocolate, which is a source of dietary magnesium, albeit a poor one. I have found that many chocoholics can easily resist chocolate binges after commencing a magnesium supplement. Magnesium deficiency will also predispose you to muscular cramps, palpitations, anxiety, insomnia, high blood pressure and migraine headaches. In particular migraine headaches can often be prevented by taking a daily magnesium supplement (approximately 400mg of elemental magnesium daily is required). For more information see my book *Magnesium – The Miracle Mineral – You won't believe the difference it makes to your health and your sex life*

Chromium and Iron

Other important minerals that help to relieve PMS symptoms are chromium and iron. These are helpful for women with heavy menstrual bleeding, fatigue and unstable blood sugar levels, which cause light headedness and sugar cravings, particularly if a meal is missed. If you have heavy menstrual bleeding, ask your doctor to order a lab test called serum iron studies – you may get a shock to find that you have a serious iron deficiency. Iron deficiency is the most common cause of fatigue in women. You will be pleased to know that this heavy bleeding can be greatly reduced with natural progesterone and an iron supplement. Iron should be taken with Vitamin C or citrus fruits to improve its absorption. An iron supplement should be taken by all women with heavy menstrual bleeding.

Essential Fatty Acids

Dietary essential fatty acids are the building blocks for a very powerful group of hormone-like chemicals in our body called *prostaglandins*. Prostaglandins regulate many vital body functions such as hormone production, circulation, immune function and inflammation, just to name a few.

It is helpful for you to know that there are three different families of prostaglandins and the prostaglandin 2 family promotes inflammation and pain, whereas the prostaglandin 1 and prostaglandin 3 families reduce inflammation and pain. (At least, it's 2 to 1 in favor of the good guys). See *Table 1* to see what foods provide you with certain essential fatty acids, which in turn are used to manufacture prostaglandins in your body.

Doctors frequently prescribe the powerful anti-prostaglandin drugs also known as non-steroidal anti-inflammatory drugs (NSAIDs). These NSAIDs suppress production in the body of all three families of prostaglandins (good and bad alike) and that is why there are sometimes side effects from these drugs. Examples of these drugs are Indocid, Nurofen, Naprogesic and Ponstan and they can be very effective in stopping the pain and inflammation of headaches, arthritis and period pains.

I have found that in many cases of PMS, headaches or painful periods, it is possible to rebalance the three prostaglandin families simply by changing the diet and taking supplements of essential fatty acids. This reduces pain and inflammation in a natural way.

To reduce the amounts of the undesirable prostaglandin 2 family you should reduce your intake of the unhealthy fats found in very fatty meats, deep fried foods and processed foods.

To increase the production of the desirable prostaglandin 1 and prostaglandin 3 families, you should consume a diet that is high in raw seeds, sprouts, raw nuts, vegetables, fish, fish oil, ground flaxseeds and cold pressed olive oil.

Supplements of fish oil, ground flaxseeds and their oil and blackcurrant seed oil will increase the production of the desirable prostaglandin 3 family, which is helpful in reducing many PMS type symptoms.

Another efficient way to balance the prostaglandin families is to take supplements of essential fatty acids. Evening primrose oil (EPO) contains the essential fatty acids linoleic acid and gamma linolenic acid (GLA). EPO will increase the prostaglandin 1 family and can be effective in reducing premenstrual headaches, breast tenderness, period pains and other symptoms of PMS.

My sister, Madeleine, an actress, finds a combination of flaxseed oil, fish oil and evening primrose oil superb for her hair and skin, and says that she is happy to go without several of life's little luxuries provided she can have her essential oils.

Table 1

Foods	Essential Fatty Acids	Prostaglandin Family	Effect in Body
Sesame seeds, sunflower seeds, raw nuts, cold pressed vegetable oils, blackcurrant seeds and their oil, evening primrose oil and borage oil	Linoleic acid Gamma linolenic acid	Prostaglandin 1 (desirable)	Reduces pain and inflammation
Saturated fats in fatty meats or preserved meats, deep-fried foods and processed foods	Arachidonic acid	Prostaglandin 2 (undesirable)	Increases pain and inflammation; can result in sticky platelets and poor circulation
Ground flaxseeds (linseeds) or their cold pressed oil, blackcurrant seed oil, fish oil and fish from cold deep oceans (mackerel, sardines, tuna, salmon), chia seeds and walnuts Note: Canned fish is acceptable	Alpha linolenic acid Eicosapentaenoic acid (EPA) Docosahexaenoic acid (DHA)	Prostaglandin 3 (desirable)	Reduces pain and inflammation

4. The Anti-PMS Diet – Golden Rules

There are a few golden rules to follow and if you observe them six days a week, you will be able to enjoy the occasional indiscretion without problems.

Golden Rules and the Good Effects

Rule: *Avoid refined carbohydrates, soft drinks and refined sugars. Get your sugar from fresh fruits.*

Effect: This aids weight control and stabilizes blood sugar levels.

Rule: *Reduce unhealthy fats, eg very fatty meats, sausages, preserved meats or deep-fried foods, processed and take away meals, ice cream and processed hydrogenated vegetable oils.*

Effect: This aids weight control, reduces hormonal imbalances, reduces cysts in the breasts and ovaries, reduces the risk of cancer and reduces inflammation and pain.

Rule: *Reduce caffeine, sugar and alcohol.*

Effect: This reduces anxiety and mood changes, fluid retention, headaches, and breast pain and breast cysts.

Rule: *Increase foods high in magnesium and iron, eg whole grains, green leafy vegetables, beetroot, unprocessed cereals, legumes, nuts, seeds, seafood and lean fresh red meat (not essential if you are vegetarian). Tahini and culinary seaweeds (such as kelp, arame, dulse, wakame) are excellent sources of trace minerals and calcium. These seaweeds or sea vegetables can be used in soups, stir fries or salads.*

Effect: This reduces headaches and increases energy levels. Prevents iron deficiency anemia. Increases bone density. Supports the function of the thyroid gland.

Rule: *Eat more frequent meals (ideally 3 meals daily) containing first class protein, eg organic eggs, organic poultry, seafood, lean fresh meat, white colored cheeses, plain acidophilus yogurt and whey protein powder. Feta or Parmesan cheese provides high quality protein and calcium. An excellent source of first class protein and fiber is obtained by combining three of the following at one meal - grains, nuts, seeds and legumes.*

Effect: This stabilizes blood sugar levels, prevents sugar and junk food binges, and increases energy levels. Reduces insulin resistance (Syndrome X) thus aiding weight loss by enhancing fat burning.

Rule: *Consume foods high in phyto-estrogens such as seeds, legumes, whole ground flaxseed and sprouts.*

Effect: This reduces hormonal imbalances and reduces the risk of hormone dependent cancers.

Rule: *Consume foods high in organic sulfur, such as the cruciferous vegetables (broccoli, cauliflower, Brussels sprouts, cabbage, kale, bok choy) and the onion family (onions of all types, leeks), garlic and organic eggs.*

Effect: The sulfur in these foods supports the detoxification pathways in the liver, which break down excess levels of estrogens and toxic chemicals that increase hormonal imbalances.

Can Lifestyle Changes Help PMS?

A reasonably healthy lifestyle is a must if you are serious about beating PMS. Let's check out the benefits of some good habits.

The tools of a healthy diet, lifestyle and nutritional supplements will provide relief for the majority of women with mild to moderate PMS. Patience and persistence are vital, as with most types of nutritional medicine, there is a time lapse of six to eight weeks before major improvements are attained.

Lifestyle and the Benefits

Lifestyle: *A regular exercise programme, including some aerobic exercise, some muscle building and relaxing exercises.*

Benefit: This reduces muscle spasm and tension. Increases brain endorphins, which are natural euphoric substances. Improves the blood supply to the hormonal glands.

Lifestyle: *Quit smoking.*

Benefit: Nicotine constricts blood vessels and reduces the blood supply to the hormonal glands, brain and the skin. Giving up smoking will increase the hormone output from your ovaries thus slowing down the ageing process. Hypnosis is very effective for quitting smoking.

Lifestyle: *Increase water intake to 70 ounces (2 liters) daily and make yourself raw vegetable and fruit juices. The best things to include in your juice are ginger, carrot, apple, citrus, cabbage and green leafy herbs such as basil, cilantro, mint and parsley.*

Benefit: This aids weight control and reduces headaches. Greatly improves the condition of the skin and hair. Reduces breast pain and period pain. Increases energy levels and improves mental clarity.

Lifestyle: *Reduce alcohol intake especially during the two premenstrual weeks.*

Benefit: This avoids embarrassing moments. There is a reduced tolerance to alcohol premenstrually with higher blood alcohol levels being attained quickly. Your moods will be much better and far more stable bringing greater self control. Tyrosine supplements can help you to quit alcohol – the powder form of tyrosine works better.

5. What Risk Factors Increase Your Chance of PMS?

1. Family History

You won't thank your ancestors for this familial trait but there is no doubt that if your mother, sisters or maternal or paternal grandmother or great grandmothers had PMS; then you are also more prone to suffer with PMS.

2. Hormonal Triggers

Many women first notice PMS after ceasing the oral contraceptive pill, after pregnancy, after postnatal depression or after miscarriage or after a tubal ligation (surgical sterilization).

Some women get awful *PMS type symptoms*, such as depression and irritability while taking the oral contraceptive pill (OCP). This is because the synthetic progesterone in the OCP reduces the production of natural progesterone from the ovaries and also blocks the hormone receptors on the cells from natural hormones.

3. Stress

PMS may appear for the first time or become much worse, after severe or prolonged stress, such as relationship difficulties, financial problems or unwanted pregnancies. Stress affects the function of the hypothalamus and the adrenal glands and this in turn imbalances the function of the ovaries.

4. Increasing Age

Typically PMS worsens during the 30s, peaking in the mid to late 30s. During the 40s, PMS becomes intertwined with the hormonal deficiencies characteristic of the premenopausal years. As a woman approaches menopause the number of follicles (eggs) in her ovaries is declining rapidly and this causes more severe deficiencies and/or imbalances of estrogen and progesterone.

5. Being a 21st Century Woman

Today's woman has, on average, two children and spends the rest of her life having regular menstrual cycles with approximately 350 to 400 menstrual periods in her reproductive life span. Therefore, if she is susceptible, she could have 350 to 400 episodes of PMS in her lifetime. Before contraception was available, a woman had around ten pregnancies, each followed by one to two years of breast feeding. Our great grandmothers usually only menstruated for two to five years out of their whole life span. Thus, as far as Mother Nature is concerned, it would seem that women are not meant to have periods and PMS, and that they are indeed designed to have more pregnancies. Biologically we are meant to be *pregnant and barefoot in the kitchen* but sociologically those days are gone for good! The price we pay is that of progesterone deficiency.

Is there a Test for PMS?

The most accurate way to determine if you have PMS is to keep a menstrual calendar on which you chart the timing of your symptoms and menstrual bleeding. It is not only the type of symptoms that is important, but rather the fact that your symptoms recur every month, sometime after ovulation. These symptoms are relieved when menstrual bleeding is established.

Maggie's chart in the next section illustrates a classic tale of PMS. There is a chart for you to print out and use to write your own symptoms at www.liverdoctor.com/progesterone. Keep your chart accurately for three months and then take it along to your doctor to enable a correct diagnosis of your hormonal imbalance. You may also send your menstrual calendar to my Health Advisory Service at PO Box 689 Camden NSW 2570 Australia or email it to ehelp@liverdoctor.com

Generally speaking, to diagnose PMS, blood and/or salivary tests to measure hormone levels are not necessary. However, if your doctor is unsure of the diagnosis, or if a serious hormonal imbalance is suspected, then blood tests are vitally important.

It is best to measure the hormone levels in the blood when you feel at your worst, as determined by your menstrual calendar. This will pinpoint exactly what type of hormonal imbalance you could have. The best time to measure progesterone levels in the blood is on day 21 of the menstrual cycle. Day one is the first day of menstrual bleeding.

Your Own Menstrual Calendar

On this chart mark the days of menstrual bleeding with an 'M' and the days of your MOST IMPORTANT SYMPTOMS with an appropriate symbol, eg:

H	=	headache
B	=	bloatedness/water retention
BT	=	breast tenderness
D	=	depression
I	=	irritability
P	=	period pains

Or invent symbols for your priority symptoms. Even if you are not menstruating, (e.g. you have had a hysterectomy), it will help your doctor if you chart the dates of your symptoms. There is an example at the end of this chapter.

The Story of Paula

In its most severe manifestation, the premenstrual syndrome is a disorder that can ruin your life. This was brought home to me one day by a 42 year old librarian called Paula, who came to see me as her last hope. Paula had first noticed severe mood changes before menstruation, shortly after an early puberty at the age of 10. By the age of 18, her premenstrual depression was so severe that she attempted suicide with an overdose of her mother's sedatives. She was diagnosed as manic-depressive and prescribed the drug Lithium. This reduced her mood swings but she still felt unwell with headaches, bloating, sore breasts and extreme fatigue for ten days before her menstrual bleeding. Paula was gradually taken off Lithium so that she could become pregnant and by the third month of her pregnancy, she felt wonderful. She said "For the first time in my life, I feel in control, peaceful and free of headaches and I love the feeling of those huge amounts of hormones filling up my body". Paula had a natural birth and things were going well until two weeks after childbirth, when severe postnatal depression began. Paula again attempted suicide and was again prescribed Lithium. Twelve months later at the age of 31, Paula, terrified of another episode of postnatal depression, begged for sterilization by having her tubes tied (tubal ligation). After consulting six gynecologists, the tubal ligation was unfortunately performed and, not surprisingly, she then began to experience severe PMS. For twelve days before every period, she felt dead and found herself in a deep pit of depression and anger. Her head ached, her abdomen swelled and she became aggressive with her husband and child. Paula felt trapped knowing that every month after ovulation she would feel as if a switch inside her brain turned on producing volcanic changes in her personality and body. Once her menstrual bleeding started, the switch would be turned off and the depression, aggression and headaches would miraculously vanish. After menstruation she felt in control but was haunted by feelings of remorse and guilt for the disruption she had caused. Her husband could recognize the night and day effect caused by this hormonal switch and he could see that she needed help. Subsequently Paula visited eight different gynecologists and tried diuretics, sedatives, anti-depressants, the oral contraceptive pill, synthetic progesterone, psychotherapy and chiropractic treatment. In a desperate attempt to save her marriage, she asked for a hysterectomy. She also complained of period pains and reluctantly, feeling that she had tried all possible therapies, her last doctor removed her uterus.

Paula felt much better for three months after her hysterectomy until during the fourth month she noticed that her depression and anger returned for two weeks. For the next six months, she found that for two weeks out of every four weeks, she was again in the grip of severe mood changes. She returned to the doctor begging to have her ovaries removed. Thankfully, this time the doctor refused and referred her to a psychiatrist.

Paula had classic PMS in a severe degree and was in urgent need of natural hormone therapy. Her hysterectomy had relieved her period pains and headaches but had done nothing to quell the cyclical surges and falls of sex hormones from her ovaries. She felt great when her ovaries were pumping out estrogen and progesterone and terrible when they stopped. Paula's case supports the research finding that when the uterus is removed and the ovaries are left in place, the symptoms and hormonal changes of PMS may persist, although often to a much lesser degree. (Ref 2).

I suggested to Paula that she would feel more emotionally stable if we maintained a steady and adequate level of natural progesterone in her blood every day. She willingly accepted an initial course of a lozenge (troche) containing a combination of natural estriol 1mg and natural progesterone 200mg. Two months after commencing the troches, Paula felt stable and happy again and remarked that the constant hormone levels in her blood provided by her troches made her feel the way she felt during pregnancy. Paula could now cope and her daily life was much easier. She felt as if a prison door had been unlocked and she would no longer be trapped in a vicious hormone cycle. Such can be the drama of severe PMS.

Women are 'hormonal creatures', riding upon the waves of hormonal surges and indeed this is largely responsible for the alluring mystery that womanhood presents to males. However for a significant percentage of women, the price of this hormonal uniqueness is too much to pay.

Thankfully, we no longer have to be victims of erratic hormonal imbalances as modern day hormonal therapy can re-program our hormonal cycle. One could say the self-programmable bionic woman has arrived!

Maggie's Menstrual Calendar

Day	January	February	March	April
1		H B D	M	
2	B	M P	M	
3	B	M P	M	
4	B	M		
5	H B D	M		
6	H B D	M		
7	H B D			
8	M P			
9	M P			
10	M			
11	M			
12	M			D
13				B D
14				B D
15				B D
16				B D
17				H B D
18				M P
19				M
20			D	M
21			B D	M
22		D	B D	M
23		B D	H B D	
24		H B D	H B D	
25		H B D	M P	
26		H B D	M P	
27	B	M P	M	
28	B	M	M	
29	B D		M	
30	H B D			
31	H B D			

6. Hormonal treatment for PMS

In cases of PMS that do not respond to nutritional supplements and exercise, corrective hormonal therapy usually works well. If PMS is so severe that it is associated with uncontrollable mood changes, reduced ability to function, thoughts of suicide, marital disruption, child abuse or dangerous behavior, then antidepressant drugs (such as the serotonin-reuptake inhibitors), as well as hormonal therapy, are usually required to restore equanimity. Many of these women have been offered sedatives and counseling and come along to the doctor desperately hoping that hormonal help will be at hand. Thankfully, it is, and it can be dramatically effective.

Progesterone –the calm, happy hormone

Progesterone is a sex hormone that is made by the female ovaries during the latter half of the menstrual cycle and in vast amounts by the placenta during pregnancy. Progesterone exerts a calming effect and can promote emotional contentment and stability. The brain has receptors for progesterone and this is why natural hormones can be so beneficial for emotional disorders.

If you find that your mood lowers during the one to two weeks before your menstrual bleeding commences, then you will probably benefit from natural progesterone. Progesterone deficiency is very common in women today because they often delay pregnancy to later in life and have fewer pregnancies. Progesterone deficiency can cause unpleasant moods such as anxiety, irritability, irrational thinking and depression. Progesterone deficiency can also cause physical health problems such as heavy and/or painful menstrual bleeding, endometriosis, fibroids, increased risk of cancer, premenstrual headaches, polycystic ovarian syndrome and unexplained infertility.

Progesterone

The use of natural progesterone was first advocated back in the 1960s by Dr Katharina Dalton, an English physician who was somewhat of a 'PMS Guru'. Dr Dalton dedicated her life to helping women with hormonal imbalances and her research and books have shown natural progesterone to be effective in relieving many types of PMS. (Ref 3, 4, 5).

Natural progesterone can be very useful in reducing the following problems, which may occur, or become much worse, during the premenstrual phase of the monthly cycle –

- Depression, anxiety and mood changes
- Fatigue
- Low blood sugar levels
- Heavy menstrual bleeding
- Iron deficiency and/or anemia
- Menstrual pain
- Pelvic congestion, pain and bloating
- Breast pain
- Migraines
- Premenstrual epilepsy
- Premenstrual asthma
- Insomnia
- Endometriosis

It is important to realize that Dr. Dalton recommended the use of natural progesterone only, which has a chemical structure identical to the progesterone produced by the ovaries. Natural progesterone is made in the laboratory from the plant hormone called diosgenin found in soybeans and sweet potatoes (yams). Because natural progesterone is identical to the progesterone produced by the ovaries it is called a *bio-identical hormone.*

Unfortunately, for PMS sufferers, doctors often prescribe strong synthetic progesterones called *progestogens*, mistakenly believing that they will have the same effect as natural progesterone. This is not true and synthetic progesterone will usually make many of the symptoms of PMS much worse. Many of these synthetic progestogens are derived from male (testosterone-like) synthetic hormones and so may cause side effects such as increased appetite, depression, irritability, weight gain, fluid retention, acne, greasy skin and increased cholesterol. These synthetic progestogen hormones attach onto the natural progesterone receptors found throughout the body and brain, but they cannot switch on all these receptors. Only natural progesterone can turn on ALL the progesterone receptors just as a key turns and releases a lock. So you can understand that synthetic progestogens will not have the same beneficial effect as natural progesterone and indeed many PMS sufferers feel more depressed and tired when they take them. However synthetic progestogens are effective at reducing heavy menstrual bleeding and some types of gynecological problems such as endometriosis.

Natural progesterone is not as effective if taken by mouth (orally), as after its absorption from the intestines, it is partially destroyed by the liver enzymes.

Therefore natural progesterone is best administered by routes that bypass the liver such as -

- Creams – which may be rubbed into the skin (transdermal) or inserted high up into the vagina
- Vaginal pessaries or suppositories

Natural progesterone can also be given in the form of lozenges known as *troches*, which are NOT designed to be sucked or chewed or swallowed. Theoretically the troche is held between the upper gum and the cheek until it is completely absorbed, with the hormone it contains being transferred directly into the bloodstream across the mucous lining of the oral cavity.

Natural progesterone can also be administered in the form of capsules, which contain tiny (micronized) particles of progesterone. Theoretically these tiny particles of progesterone are more resistant to breakdown by the enzymes in the gut and the liver, so that more progesterone gets into the bloodstream.

By giving natural progesterone in these ways, we are aiming to bypass the liver so that the progesterone can be absorbed directly into the circulation and carried to the progesterone receptors on your cells.

How to use progesterone for PMS

Generally natural progesterone therapy is started five days after the end of your menstrual bleeding and this allows for several days before the expected onset of PMS symptoms. The progesterone is then continued daily up to the first day of menstrual bleeding. Once the bleeding starts the progesterone should be stopped. If you find it difficult to judge when to begin using the progesterone, you can start it at the time of ovulation, which is normally 14 days before the expected onset of your menstrual bleeding. Make sure you stop the progesterone on the first day of your menstrual bleeding and this way the progesterone is fitting in with your own natural menstrual cycle.

Each PMS sufferer is an individual and trial and error using different dosages, forms and schedules of progesterone may be required before the symptoms are fully under control. My personal preference is to administer natural progesterone in the form of a cream, which is rubbed into the skin of the inner upper arms or the inner upper thighs. You should apply the cream to dry skin after your shower, and if you shower or bathe twice daily, then it may be more effective to apply the cream twice daily after each shower. The cream needs to be rubbed very thoroughly into the skin so that the entire amount is well absorbed into the skin, with no cream remaining visible or detectable on the skin. Some doctors are very cynical about the use of creams containing natural progesterone because they do not believe that the progesterone is effectively absorbed through the skin in to the bloodstream. In other words they do not think that clinically effective amounts of progesterone can be achieved in the body by using the creams. However a study published in the American Journal of Obstetrics and Gynecology in 1999, found that absorption of progesterone from creams was just as good as absorption of estrogen from patches. They concluded that the application of progesterone cream to the skin appeared to be a safe and effective route of administration.(Ref 9)

Note:

- Progesterone cream is not a contraceptive and indeed will increase fertility!
- Natural progesterone does not work if you are taking the oral contraceptive pill.

Progesterone deficiency is common in:

- Young women with menstrual problems, including teenagers
- Women after childbirth where it may be associated with postnatal depression

- Women with cyclical mood disorders
- Women with thyroid problems such as Hashimoto's thyroiditis or Grave's disease or multi-nodular goiter
- Women after miscarriage
- Peri-menopausal women
- Women with autoimmune disease

How do I know if I am progesterone deficient?

It is not generally necessary or useful to do blood or salivary tests to prove that a deficiency of progesterone exists. This is because a doctor who understands progesterone can tell from the history of the patient if they are deficient. A woman who is progesterone deficient will have several of the symptoms below and hopefully her doctor will recognize she is deficient. However it is not uncommon for the patient to teach the doctor about natural progesterone and have to ask for it herself!

Symptoms of progesterone deficiency can include:

- Heavy periods
- Painful periods
- Endometrial hyperplasia (overgrowth or excessive thickness of the uterine lining)
- Premenstrual headaches
- Fibroids or adenomyosis of the uterus
- Endometriosis
- Unexplained infertility
- Polycystic ovarian syndrome
- Premenstrual syndrome/moodiness
- Postnatal depression
- Worsening of thyroid conditions
- Iron deficiency
- Infrequent or irregular periods
- Hair loss
- Worsening of autoimmune diseases

- Breast pain
- Breast lumpiness
- Osteoporosis
- Insomnia

Keeping a menstrual calendar of your symptoms to show your doctor can help to pinpoint the premenstrual exacerbation.

The good news is that natural progesterone therapy can often alleviate these symptoms in women of all ages. Natural progesterone is safe to use in women of all ages - from early teens to post menopausal women, it can relieve symptoms of hormonal imbalance.

Thus one would think that natural progesterone is commonly prescribed for these diverse and common problems. In reality few doctors prescribe natural progesterone. Natural progesterone cannot be patented; thus drug companies do not promote it or educate doctors about its use or benefits. This is a pity and results in much unneeded suffering.

In my opinion, the best way to administer natural progesterone is in the form of a cream which is rubbed into the skin. The cream can be used once or twice daily and required doses range from 20mg to 400mg daily. The average doses are 50 to 100mg daily. In Australia you will need a doctor's prescription for natural progesterone and it is made up into a cream by a compounding pharmacist. In the USA a prescription is not needed although this may change. For more information contact my Women's Health Advisory Service in the USA on 623 334 3232 or 02 4655 8855 in Australia or email ehelp@liverdoctor.com

Is natural progesterone safe?

Natural progesterone is very safe and is usually free of side effects. If excess doses of progesterone are used, the only side effects are abdominal bloating, breakthrough bleeding, constipation and feeling too relaxed or sleepy.

These side effects can be eliminated by reducing the dose. Pure natural progesterone does not cause birth defects or harm to the fetus if you become pregnant, and indeed will reduce your chances of miscarriage. If you do fall pregnant whilst taking progesterone, continue to use it for the first 2 to 3 months of pregnancy, but you should notify your doctor if you are using progesterone once you fall pregnant.

To read a scientific debate on the safety of bioidentical hormones visit https://www.sandracabot.com/bioidentical-hormone-debate

Progesterone can balance excess estrogen

Progesterone is needed to balance the effects of estrogen. Estrogen causes the cells lining the uterus to divide and grow, whereas progesterone inhibits this growth. Estrogen can be described as a fertilizer, and progesterone as the lawn mower. Thus progesterone is needed to oppose the stimulatory effects of estrogen on the uterus.

The mechanisms that progesterone uses to keep estrogen in check are –

• Progesterone reduces estrogen's stimulating effects upon cancer-promoting genes.

• Progesterone promotes the conversion of the stronger estradiol to the weaker type of estrogen called estrone.

• Progesterone reduces the number of estrogen receptors on the cells, thus reducing the sensitivity of the cells to estrogen.

These are all very important balancing actions, and this vital role of progesterone explains why all women who are given estrogen, should always be given progesterone (preferably the natural form), even if they have had a hysterectomy. Natural progesterone is also needed for healthy bone tissue, probably because it stimulates the bone building cells called osteoblasts.

Progesterone is only produced from the ovaries after ovulation. Disorders of ovulation are common, and many women ovulate only irregularly, infrequently or rarely, especially if they have polycystic ovarian syndrome (PCOS) or as they approach the premenopausal years. The most common cause of infrequent or absent ovulation in premenopausal women, is polycystic ovarian syndrome. See the case history of Georgina later in this book. In premenopausal women who have ovulation problems, we find that estrogen is produced from the ovary, but there is no progesterone, or only inadequate amounts of progesterone are produced. The amounts of progesterone are insufficient to balance the estrogen – this causes the situation of unopposed estrogen.

This unopposed estrogen will stimulate the lining of the uterus to grow too thick, and the lack of progesterone means that the lining can become abnormally thick – this is called endometrial hyperplasia. Women with endometrial hyperplasia often complain of very heavy menstrual bleeding with large clots. If this hyperplasia becomes chronic, precancerous changes may occur in the cells lining the uterus – this is called atypical hyperplasia. Around 20% of women with atypical hyperplasia will go on to get uterine cancer, if this problem is not treated. By administering progesterone (natural or synthetic), we are able to prevent, or even reverse, endometrial hyperplasia. Thus progesterone has an anti-cancer effect. If you have very heavy menstrual bleeding, especially if it is erratic or irregular in timing, you must see a gynecologist for a dilatation and curettage of the uterine lining. The gynecologist will also examine the lining of your uterus with a flexible telescopic device called a hysteroscope to check for any abnormal growths which could signal cancer. Unfortunately too many women put up with this abnormal bleeding and develop uterine cancer, so you cannot be too careful here.

A study published in *The Journal of the Climacteric and Postmenopause, Maturitas 20 (1995) 191-198*, (Ref 12) provides convincing evidence that natural progesterone can control endometrial hyperplasia. In this study, 78 premenopausal women with endometrial hyperplasia were treated from the 10th to the 25th day of their menstrual cycle with a vaginal cream containing 100mg of natural micronized progesterone. This progesterone therapy achieved a complete regression (reversal) of the hyperplasia in 90.5% of cases. During treatment there was a significant reduction in the amount, duration and frequency of the menstrual bleeding. Other good news is that minimal side effects were observed during this trial, which is in contrast to synthetic progestogens, which commonly produce side effects.

The researchers concluded that vaginal administration of natural progesterone is –

- Effective in treating endometrial hyperplasia
- Safe to use, because it does not exert unfavorable changes on the blood levels of cholesterol

This is in contrast to synthetic progestogens, which may exert adverse changes upon the cholesterol levels.

Thus natural progesterone administered vaginally, should be considered as a serious alternative to synthetic progestogens in clinical practice, especially in women with metabolic disorders such as polycystic ovarian syndrome, Syndrome X, diabetes, hypertension, fatty liver and problems with high levels of blood fats (triglycerides and cholesterol).

Progesterone can also be given in a micronized form (ultrafine consistency), which means that the progesterone particles are much smaller; this is done to improve absorption from the gut. Micronized progesterone is administered in capsules. A dose of 200mg of micronized progesterone, given for 15 days per month, is considered equivalent to 10mg of the synthetic progestogen called Provera. If the natural progesterone is given in a dose of 100mg daily for 25 days per month, this is also considered equivalent to 10mg of Provera. Micronized progesterone was evaluated in the Postmenopausal Estrogen/Progestin Interventions (PEPI) Trial. The micronized progesterone was found to be as effective as the synthetic progestogens in opposing the effects of estrogen on the uterus. (Ref 10)

The PEPI Trial showed that 200mg of natural micronized progesterone, given for 12 days of the month, was sufficient to prevent overstimulation of the uterus by the brand of estrogen called Premarin. The micronized progesterone was shown to have a more favorable effect upon blood levels of cholesterol than the synthetic progestogens. Because natural progesterone is more effective in correcting the adverse changes that occur in cholesterol levels after the menopause, it should be safer than synthetic progestogens, when it comes to reducing the risk of heart disease.

To read a scientific debate on the safety of bioidentical hormones visit https://www.sandracabot.com/bioidentical-hormone-debate

Doctors have been educated to use synthetic progestogens in HRT for premenopausal and post-menopausal women. However now that the WHI study (Ref 11) has shown that synthetic progestogens are not desirable for long term use in HRT, many doctors will be looking towards safer solutions, such as natural progesterone. However, natural progesterone does far more than just replace the use of synthetic progestogens, and has several powerful health promoting benefits in itself.

What is the difference between natural and synthetic progesterone?

Natural progesterone has very different effects to synthetic progestogens in the body, and is far less likely to produce unpleasant side effects. For example synthetic progestogens can increase the risk of spasm in the coronary arteries, whereas natural progesterone reduces such spasms. Natural progesterone is a smooth muscle relaxant and thus usually helps to reduce menstrual cramps. Synthetic progestogens are far more likely to produce side effects such as weight gain, depression, fluid retention, headaches and breast tenderness. This is because the synthetic progestogens increase the workload of the liver, as they must be broken down by the detoxification pathways (cytochrome P-450 enzymes) in the liver.

7. Different ways to use Natural Progesterone

Natural Progesterone Cream

Natural progesterone can be administered as a cream applied to the skin of the inner upper arms or inner upper legs. The cream can also be inserted high up into the vagina last thing at night on retiring to bed.

The average dosage is 50mg daily but the dose may range from 10mg to 200mg daily. It is commenced approximately 14 days before onset of the menstrual bleeding is due.

The benefits of natural progesterone are relief of the symptoms of the premenstrual syndrome such as mood disorders, pelvic congestion, migraines, breast pain, heavy bleeding, menstrual pain and fatigue. Progesterone often alleviates postnatal depression.

Possible side effects include some breakthrough bleeding if doses are excessive. Breakthrough bleeding is more likely to occur if the cream is inserted high up in the vagina. When used vaginally, some vaginal irritation may occur if the base of the cream is unsuitable. If the progesterone cream causes vaginal irritation, speak to your compounding pharmacists about changing the base of the cream. Excessive doses of progesterone can lead to bloating and drowsiness. If you have any of the side effects, reduce the dose until the side effects disappear. As you can see the required dose can vary a lot, as every PMS sufferer is an individual, and by experimenting with the dose of the cream you can avoid any nuisance side effects.

Natural Progesterone Vaginal Pessaries

A pessary is an oval shaped condensed solid form of progesterone which is inserted high into the vagina. These can be made up by a compounding pharmacist in doses varying from 20 to 200mg per pessary. Vaginal pessaries of progesterone are often used in infertility clinics to increase fertility and to reduce the risk of early miscarriage. They can be used to relieve symptoms of the PMS and also reduce heavy menstrual bleeding and menstrual pain.

Natural Progesterone Injections

Natural progesterone may also be administered by oily depot injections given into the fatty areas of the buttocks. The dosage is 25 to 100mg daily given for the 14 days before menstrual bleeding.

The benefits include the relief of the symptoms of the premenstrual syndrome such as mood disorders, pelvic congestion, migraines, heavy bleeding, menstrual pain and fatigue. The injections can also be used to relieve postnatal depression. Because the injections are oily they act as a slow release depot of progesterone. Possible side effects are tenderness and lumpiness in the buttocks, breakthrough bleeding and fluid retention. I have not used progesterone injections for several years now because of these possible side effects and I find women prefer the progesterone creams, capsules or troches.

Natural Progesterone Troches

Natural Progesterone troches are lozenges that are placed between the upper gum and the cheek. They slowly dissolve through the mucous membrane of the cheek and the progesterone is absorbed directly into the circulation. Do not suck, chew or swallow the lozenges. They come in a variety of flavors. Capsules containing micronized progesterone can be swallowed.

The average dose of natural progesterone is 50mg daily but the dose may range from 25 to 400mg daily. It needs to be given for the 14 days before menstrual bleeding commences.

The benefits of the troches is the relief of the symptoms of the premenstrual syndrome such as mood disorders, pelvic congestion, migraines, heavy bleeding, menstrual pain and fatigue. May reduce breast pain. May increase fertility. May alleviate post natal depression.

If doses are excessive some breakthrough bleeding, drowsiness and fluid retention may occur. In some women the troche may produce irritation of the gum. In allergy-prone people the troches may cause allergic type symptoms such as rashes and swelling. The progesterone cream is best used in allergy-prone people. If the troches contain sugar they may increase dental caries. If these side effects occur then reduce the dosage of hormones in the troche, or change to the progesterone cream.

Synthetic Progesterone

Synthetic progesterone (also known as progestogens) are available - common brands are norethisterone, norgesterol, and medroxy-progesterone acetate tablets. These tablets can be given every day, or for the 14 days before menstrual bleeding begins. The dosage varies depending upon the brand of tablet and the medical reason for which it is prescribed. Progestogens (*synthetic progesterones*) are effective in reducing endometriosis, heavy menstrual bleeding and endometrial hyperplasia.

These synthetic progestogens have a slightly masculine effect, which may result in weight gain, pimples, greasy skin and hair. Some brands may cause fluid retention, moodiness, depression and elevation of cholesterol. They often make depression and other mood disorders much worse.

Natural estrogen

In a small number of cases of cyclical premenstrual mood disorder, natural progesterone therapy by itself fails to relieve all the symptoms. This is more likely in older women who are premenopausal, in which case there may be a deficiency of estrogen as well as progesterone. This can be determined with blood tests to measure levels of estrogen and follicle stimulating hormone (FSH).

If your FSH levels are over 40 mIU/mL, this indicates all your ovarian follicles have been used up and thus your ovaries can no longer manufacture significant amounts of estrogen or progesterone.

In such cases the use of natural estrogen combined with the natural progesterone may break the cycle of unpleasant PMS. Some natural estrogen may also be helpful in PMS sufferers, who have undergone hysterectomy or tubal ligation, as after these operations the blood supply to the ovaries may be reduced. This may result in a reduced hormonal output from the ovaries and therefore increasing PMS.

Natural estrogens may be helpful for premenstrual syndrome and mood disorders and may improve libido. This is especially in premenopausal women or after hysterectomy where the ovaries may not work as well after surgery. Estrogens reduce vaginal dryness and vaginal discomfort and improve bladder function. Estrogens also improve skin texture and reduce acne and facial hair.

Both natural progesterone and most types of estrogen will reduce insomnia and hot flushes.

There are 3 types of natural estrogen produced by the ovaries and the fat tissue in your body; these are known as Estradiol, Estriol and Estrone with estradiol being the most potent and estriol the weakest and safest. These types of natural estrogens are called bio-identical estrogens, as they are chemically identical to the estrogens produced by your ovaries. Estrogens can be given in the form of creams, gels, troches, tablets or patches. Estrogens can be used cyclically for 2 to 3 weeks every month, or used everyday. It is important to give some form of progesterone with the estrogen and I prefer natural progesterone, as it is more effective and safer. The safest way to administer estrogen is in the form of creams or patches. The creams can be used on the outside of the vaginal opening (the vulva) to prevent dryness and restore natural lubrication. Usually only small doses of estrogen are required and I most commonly use estriol in a daily dose of 1 to 2 mg daily. A doctor's script is required for estrogens.

Other types of estrogen such as estrogen tablets or estrogen implants can be used, although they are relatively more potent and thus more likely to cause symptoms of estrogen excess (estrogen dominance).

The estrogen implants are best used in women who have had a hysterectomy, as they are relatively potent and may cause an increase in menstrual bleeding and other symptoms of estrogen dominance. Since the results of the Women's Health Initiative Study (Ref 11) were published in July 2002, all doctors have become aware that long term estrogen therapy will increase the risk of breast cancer. If the estrogen is combined with synthetic progesterone, this type of hormone therapy becomes even more risky to use long term with an increased risk of blood clots and strokes. Thus it is not wise to use potent forms of estrogen therapy for many years, and this means that estrogen implants are really only suitable for short term use. This means for not more than one year.

If you find that you need to take some form of estrogen to obtain relief from your hormonal symptoms, I suggest that you stick to the estrogen creams or patches, as the doses used can be much smaller and easily fine tuned to provide the smallest possible dose that relieves your symptoms. It is important to check the results of the estrogen therapy with regular blood or salivary estrogen levels, and suitable intervals are every 3 months initially and thereafter every 6 to 12 months. If you have your hormone levels tested every month you may have to pay for it yourself, as Medicare may find this excessive.

In my experience I have found that estrogen implants can result in very high blood levels of estrogen being found on blood tests. This would be worrying if women decided to continue with this potent form of estrogen for many years. In contrast I have found that when using small doses of natural hormones in the form of creams, the blood levels of estrogen, progesterone and testosterone stay within safe and very modest levels.

Some women find that they only need to use the natural estrogen during the 14 days preceding menstrual bleeding, whereas others may feel more in balance if they use the estrogen every day. In women who still have a uterus, the use of natural estrogen must be balanced with progesterone.

Excessive doses or the more potent forms of estrogen are best avoided, as they can lead to symptoms of estrogen dominance.

Estrogen dominance symptoms can include –

• Breast pain and lumpiness
• Fluid retention
• Gallstones
• Heavy or painful menstrual bleeding
• Increased size of fibroids
• Migraine headaches
• Aching legs
• Blood clots
• Weight gain in the hips and thighs

If these side effects occur you will need your doctor to reduce the dosage of estrogen, or change to the weakest form of estrogen which is estriol. It is safer to avoid potent forms of estrogen (such as implants, injections and tablets) and use estrogen creams or patches instead. If this does not work, stop the estrogen and use natural progesterone only.

The Oral Contraceptive Pill (OCP)

There are many types of OCPs and the best types for PMS contain the estrogen called ethinylestradiol combined with a friendly or neutral progestogen such as gestodene or desogestrel. The OCP is supplied as either a 21 day or 28 day packet of tablets. The primary use of OCPs is to provide contraception, but if you have PMS, it's important to use an OCP that contains neutral progestogens such as gestodene or desogestrel. The stronger synthetic progestogens, such as norethisterone or norgestrel, tend to cause moodiness, aggression and weight gain, and are best avoided if you have PMS.

The OCP can be helpful for PMS, especially if you need contraception, but it is usually not nearly as effective as natural progesterone. The OCP suppresses ovulation, which may help some women with premenstrual mood disorder. The OCP can relieve some types of period pain and reduce heavy bleeding. The OCP provides very good contraception, unlike natural progesterone, which actually increases fertility in many women!

Possible side effects of the OCP include –

- Migraine headaches, which can be severe
- Nausea and gallstones
- Fluid retention
- Weight gain and bloating
- Reduced or total loss of sex drive
- Breast pain and lumpiness
- Blood clots and aggravation of varicose veins
- Elevation of blood pressure
- Moodiness and depression in susceptible women
- Increased risk of strokes

If the OCP gives you side effects, you will need to experiment with your doctor to try different brands of the OCP, as they contain different types of hormones. All the hormones used in the OCP are synthetic and some women will be unable to tolerate the side effects.

In women with very heavy menstrual bleeding, a contraceptive intra-uterine device called the Mirena can work effectively to reduce the menstrual bleeding to very light or absent. The Mirena does not usually help to overcome PMS symptoms such as mood disorder and in such cases the natural progesterone cream can be used with the Mirena. This is quite safe and does not interfere with the contraceptive efficiency of the Mirena.

Note: Some injections are called Depot Injections; this means they slowly release their hormones from an oily base and are thus long acting injections lasting from 14 to 90 days.

Note: It is imperative that women who wish to avoid pregnancy and are taking drugs or hormones to treat PMS have adequate means of contraception.

Antidepressant drugs

In cases of severe premenstrual depression, menopausal depression or postnatal depression, an antidepressant drug may need to be used along with the progesterone. The serotonin re-uptake inhibitor drugs, also known as SSRIs, have been shown to prevent premenstrual mood disorder and are generally very safe and effective. The original SSRI drug discovered in the late 1980s was called Prozac and revolutionized the medical specialty of psychiatry. Today there are many different brands of SSRI drugs such as Lovan, Citalopram, Aropax, Efexor and Zoloft etc. and they all work by increasing levels of serotonin in the brain. This prevents the drop in serotonin levels in the brain that occurs premenstrually in PMS sufferers.

The SSRIs may reduce libido and make it harder for women to have orgasms, which can be problematic for some women. I have found that by using natural progesterone and nutritional supplements, it is possible to use much smaller doses of SSRIs and this way we can often avoid side effects. Unless natural progesterone and nutritional supplements are used, many sufferers of severe PMS find that they need increasing doses of SSRIs, or indeed that the SSRIs stop working.

Case history of Georgina

Georgina came to my medical practice one day as a new patient and her story has really stuck in my mind. She plonked herself in the chair on the other side of my desk and looked tired and distraught. I asked her "why have you come to see me today?". She replied "I am sick of lying in bed at night and thinking of 27 ways to kill my husband".

Unfortunately she was not joking and had really come to the end of the road, so to speak. I think she saw me as the last resort and thankfully I was able to relive her suffering. Georgina had all the classic symptoms of polycystic ovarian syndrome (PCOS) – she was overweight, apple shaped (android body type) and had not had a menstrual period for 2 years. She was aged 39 so her lack of regular menstrual bleeding was abnormal, considering she was not menopausal.

Blood tests on Georgina revealed that her levels of male hormones (androgens) were very high and her progesterone levels were very low. She also had high blood levels of insulin and was pre-diabetic. Georgina had been on SSRI antidepressant drugs for 2 years and they were no longer controlling her depression and aggressive moods. This poor lady had hormones more like that of a man and really needed progesterone. I prescribed natural progesterone cream 100mg daily and 2 weeks later Georgina had a menstrual bleed – for the first time in 2 years! With the onset of the bleeding came an emotional release and a feeling of calm relaxation. I also prescribed a low carbohydrate diet free of grains and sugar and told her to follow the eating plan in my book Fatty Liver – You Can Reverse It. Georgina had a fatty liver caused from the high insulin levels due to her previously high carbohydrate diet. Her poor liver function had contributed to her severe hormonal imbalance, so I also prescribed Livatone Plus™, and selenium to support her liver function.

Over the next 6 months Georgina continued to have a regular monthly menstrual cycle and lost her feelings of aggression and irritability. She felt calm and content and lost a considerable amount of weight. Her facial hair and acne also improved greatly and her sex drive returned. Luckily for her poor unsuspecting husband she no longer fantasized about ways to kill him!

Hormonal imbalances can drive women to do all sorts of extreme things premenstrually and during the postnatal period, and these things can be most out of character. Dr Katharina Dalton dedicated her life to helping women with PMS and postnatal depression and she was really the pioneer of natural progesterone therapy and wrote several books on the subject. Dr Dalton acted as an expert witness in criminal court cases trying to have the charges against women reduced because of their hormonal problems. She managed to prove that in many cases natural progesterone therapy could have prevented aggressive behavior.

8. The principles for an Anti-PMS Diet and Lifestyle

To reduce the tendency for hormonal fluctuations to upset your mental and emotional wellbeing you need to consume a diet to improve the function of your brain and nervous system

Here are a few astounding brain facts -

- Your brain is the fattiest organ in your body; indeed if you remove the water from your brain it is made of more than 60% fat.

- 75% of the weight of the brain is water – so if you don't drink enough water, don't expect your brain to work well!

- There are around 100,000 miles of blood vessels in your brain – so you need to look after your blood vessels!

- There are around 100 billion neurons in your brain – that's a lot! Consider that the world's population is 6.5 billion – no wonder you are so smart!

- Each neuron has between 1,000 to 10,000 connections to other neurons – wow that leaves the internet for dead!

- Cholesterol is a vital fat for your brain and it insulates the nerve pathways – if your brain is low in cholesterol it will function more slowly – like dial up internet and not like high speed broadband.

Healthy happy fats for the brain

Premenstrual depression and anxiety can be greatly aggravated if the diet does not provide adequate amounts of the essential fatty acids. The most important fatty acids for the brain are the omega 3 fatty acids known as EPA and DHA. The body cannot manufacture its own supply of these fatty acids – that is why they are called essential!

Studies have shown that in depressed subjects who have a poor diet devoid of, or very low in, omega 3 fatty acids, a remarkable improvement in mental and emotional health is achieved by giving supplements of fish oil. Scans of the brains of these depressed subjects showed that the size of the brain increased after giving the fish oil supplements and especially the areas of the brain concerned with emotion and memory.

I am not surprised by the findings of these studies, as when one considers what the brain is made of, it is quite logical and not unexpected. Your brain is largely made of fat, but not just any old fat! You would not want to have a brain made of margarine or cheap cooking oil! The predominant fat found in the brain is omega 3 fatty acid. There are also large amounts of pure cholesterol found in the healthy human brain. Other fats in the brain are phospholipid fats and omega 6 fatty acids. The brain is the fattiest or oiliest organ in your body and it's meant to be like that.

So if you suffer with premenstrual depression and/or anxiety or poor cognition, take a look at your diet. Do you regularly eat oily fish such as salmon, sardines, tuna, mackerel, herrings, anchovies etc? If not, then you are probably deficient in the happy omega 3 fats, which could be making you depressed.

For similar reasons I am not a fan of the low fat diet craze, as low fat diets do not supply the brain tissue with enough fat; this can increase the risk of depression, anxiety and poor memory. It has been found that very low levels of cholesterol in the blood are associated with a higher incidence of depression.

If you do not eat plenty of oily fish, I recommend fish oil supplements, ideally in a liquid form; there are lime and orange flavored liquid fish oils available. If you hate the taste of fish oil, take the capsules. Generally in depressed people I recommend 2000 to 4000mg of pure high quality fish oil daily. In those with a very poor diet, higher doses of 6000 to 8000 mg daily may be required to lift the depression.

If you keep your fish oil in the fridge and take it just before you eat, it should not cause digestive upset or an unpleasant after taste. I prefer to use the liquid forms of fish oil especially if large doses are required. This is because the large soft gelatin capsules, which contain the fish oil, may contain substances that induce allergies or digestive upsets when taken in large amounts over long periods of time. My preferred fish oil is high quality and flavored with lemon/lime oils and found in a glass bottle. If you don't like fish oil liquid, high quality capsules can be used instead. Krill oil is also a good source of omega 3 fatty acids;

however it is hard to obtain adequate amounts of omega 3 from krill because they are so small and quite expensive. Krill are tiny shrimp-like crustaceans found in the cold oceans.

If you are intolerant or allergic to fish or fish oil, you can obtain omega 3 fatty acids by taking flaxseed oil in liquid or capsule form. Make sure the flaxseed oil is of high quality and once opened it should be kept in the fridge. Generally 2000 to 4000mg daily of flaxseed oil is required; so check the label to see the amount of liquid or the number of capsules you need to take.

Some folks just hate taking oily supplements and for these people I suggest they boost their intake of omega 3 essential fatty acids by taking one to two tablespoons daily of ground whole flaxseeds. You can buy whole flaxseeds and pass them through a food processor or grinder to produce a tasty sweet flavored powder. You can also buy the flaxseed powder but make sure it looks fresh. Flaxseed powder should be kept in the fridge because fatty acids are fragile and easily become rancid; once rancid they are useless. I keep my flaxseed powder in the freezer where it stays fresh much longer. Flaxseed powder can be stirred into cereals, yogurt or smoothies and even children enjoy its sweet nutty taste. Make sure you grind the flaxseeds well into a fine powder for better absorption from the intestines. Other sources of omega 3 fats are chia seeds and walnuts. Eggs are a good source of healthy fat and protein for the brain and I recommend you eat them regularly.

Cold pressed oils such as olive oil, avocado oil, coconut oil and macadamia nut oil make tasty salad dressings and recipes and provide beneficial fats for the brain.

Protein

Every single neurotransmitter in the brain is made of protein. Neurotransmitters are the chemicals that control our moods and cognition, and transmit messages between brain cells. The most important neurotransmitters for mood, libido, motivation and memory are serotonin, dopamine and acetylcholine. You need good quality dietary protein to make neurotransmitters. Make sure you have at least three meals daily containing first class protein. They do not have to be large meals or contain large amounts of protein, but they need to supply the amino acids that the brain requires. Amino acids are the building blocks of protein and they are found in protein foods. The brain's neurotransmitters are made from amino acids.

All the amino acids essential to the manufacture of neurotransmitters are found in first class protein foods such as –

- Animal protein from foods such as eggs, poultry, dairy products, white and red meats and seafood
- Protein powder shakes, the best ones containing whey protein
- Plant protein if it is combined correctly can satisfy the brain's requirements for amino acids. You must combine 3 of the following four food groups at one meal to get all of the amino acids essential for the production of the happy chemicals required by the brain – namely legumes, nuts, seeds and grains. Legumes consist of beans, chickpeas or lentils.

Eating protein regularly prevents large fluctuations in blood sugar levels (hypoglycemia) and this has a stabilizing effect on the mood and mental energy levels.

Reduce foods high in refined sugar

Foods and beverages, such as candies, sweets, cakes, muffins, bagels, donuts and soft drinks, that contain large amounts of sugar; these should be decreased and used as occasional treats rather than regular dietary items. Too much sugar will destabilize the blood sugar levels and when the blood sugar levels drop too low, unpleasant mood changes can occur such as anxiety or depression as well as severe fatigue and headaches.

Large amounts of sugar can increase the heart rate and cause agitation and hyperstimulation of the nervous system. It is important to avoid large amounts of sugary foods before bedtime as they may cause insomnia. If you need a bed time snack try a protein food such as a piece of cheese or nuts. Many people feel much calmer and more energetic when they reduce sugary foods and increase dietary protein.

Unstable blood sugar levels can produce mental fogginess, dizziness and unpleasant moods such as anxiety and irritability. They can also lead to fatigue, sugar cravings and disturbances of appetite. Those suffering with anxiety-depression syndromes often have poor diets and consume large amounts of refined sugar and caffeine, which destabilize blood sugar levels. This can worsen their symptoms of nervous dysfunction. Eating sugar gives temporary relief from depression or anxiety, but these symptoms worsen as the blood sugar level falls again later. Supplements of the minerals chromium and magnesium can greatly reduce this problem and reduce cravings for sweets or other high carbohydrate foods.

Avoid the artificial sweetener aspartame, which is found in many diet foods and diet sodas. It is represented on labels by the food additive number 951. Aspartame is an excito-toxin that can seriously disturb function of your brain cells – for more information see www.dorway.com

Increase antioxidant foods

The brain has a high requirement for antioxidants because it is a fatty organ and as such is fragile and prone to oxidative damage from free radicals. Free radicals can attack the brain cells (neurons) causing inflammation and if this is allowed to become chronic, damage to the neurons can occur. This could reduce the ability of neurons to manufacture neurotransmitters and damage the cell membranes of the neurons, interfering with their ability to transmit messages between each other. This can result in mood changes and sluggish mental function.

Free radicals are produced in the body from stress, cigarette smoking, excess alcohol, high sugar intake, toxic chemicals, infections and pollution.

Antioxidants neutralize free radicals thereby preventing them from inflicting damage upon brain cells. When a person is under increased stress they use up antioxidants at a faster rate and they need to be replenished on a regular basis.

The most important antioxidants to protect our brain cells are –

- **Vitamin E** – found in fresh wheat germ, whole grain cereals, eggs, leafy greens, avocados and raw fresh nuts and seeds

- **Vitamin C** – found in bell peppers (capsicums), all citrus fruits, berries, kiwi fruits and many other fresh fruits
- **Selenium** – because of soil deficiencies and mass produced food (including farmed fish) it is hard to get enough selenium in your food; so a supplement of 100 to 200mcg daily is advisable. Dietary sources of selenium include Brazil nuts, broccoli, mushrooms, cabbage, onions, garlic, radishes, brewer's yeast, fish and organ meats.

Phyto-chemicals are powerful antioxidants found in fresh fruits and vegetables.

Phyto-chemicals can be found in –

Sulfur containing foods such as cruciferous vegetables (broccoli, cabbage, cauliflower, Brussels sprouts), onions, garlic, chives and radishes. They contain natural sulfur chemicals (such as glucosinolates and isothiocyanates) and these help the liver to break down toxic levels of estrogens. This reduces PMS and the risk of estrogen-induced cancers.

Green colored vegetables and fruits – these contain chlorophyll and vitamin K, which cleanse the liver and reduce excessive menstrual bleeding. They also contain folic acid which reduces depression.

Purple colored fruits and vegetables contain anthocyanidins which improve immune and liver function.

The pigments, which give fruits and vegetables their bright colors, are powerful antioxidants. Try to eat one large vegetable salad containing five different colors of vegetables daily. Also aim to eat two to three pieces of fresh fruit daily. Choose produce that is in season.

Fresh green herbs – these are very high in antioxidants and magnesium and can be used in salads or juices. It can be quite therapeutic and also fun to start a little herb garden at home to grow your own organic herbs. I suggest you grow the following – parsley, mint, basil, coriander, thyme, rosemary, shallots and garlic chives. Mint is excellent for lifting the spirits and cleansing the system. Thyme is an excellent natural antibiotic and garlic chives, coriander and basil are liver tonics.

Juice Recipe to reduce PMS

Ginger – 1/2 inch (1 cm) slice fresh root

1 carrot

2 cabbage leaves

2 oranges

1 lemon

1 cup fresh green herbs – parsley, mint, basil, cilantro etc

Pass through juicer and serve with ice cubes

Eating or juicing fresh herbs and vegetables is important for a healthy liver and improving your liver function can help to overcome Premenstrual depression and moodiness. Metaphysically speaking, the liver is *the seat of anger* so if your liver is overloaded, overworked or toxic you may feel more angry, irritable and moody. Anger turned inwards can make you depressed and many natural therapists recommend a good detox of the liver and bowels to cleanse the mind of irritant toxins. I think there is great merit in this and improving your liver function by eating more raw fresh fruits, vegetables and herbs often clears the mind as well as improving your spirits. For similar reasons you may find that a good liver tonic such as Livatone™, improves your moods.

Breast pain relief

Some women suffer from sensitive breasts during some phases of the menstrual cycle. Several nutrients, as well as lifestyle factors, can affect the health of your breast tissue. The good news is - there is a great deal you can do to protect the health of your breasts and reduce your risk of breast cancer.

Breast health recommendations –

- Have regular breast checks from your doctor and perform breast self examinations every month.
- Avoid excess alcohol intake.
- Include plenty of antioxidant rich foods in your diet, such as raw vegetables and their juices, raw fruits and white or green tea.
- Include phyto-estrogen rich foods in your diet such as nuts, seeds

and legumes (beans, peas & lentils) and ground flaxseeds.

- Keep your weight in the healthy range and exercise regularly.
- Minimize your exposure to toxic chemicals and plastics. Avoid heating food in plastic containers or plastic wraps. Don't drink hot beverages from Styrofoam cups.
- Install a water filter in your home.
- If you have lumpy breasts, it may be wise to avoid prolonged use of oral contraceptives which contain synthetic estrogens.
- Ensure you receive enough of the nutrients vital for supporting healthy breast tissue – these are Vitamin D, iodine and selenium.

Daily supplements to improve the health of your breast tissue include iodine 160 mcg, selenium100 mcg and Vitamin D3 1000 IU. For further information about help with breast pain, contact my Health Advisory Service by email at ehelp@liverdoctor.com or phone 623 334 3232 in the USA - See the book *The Breast Cancer Prevention Guide.*

9. Additional Natural Treatments for Premenstrual Depression and Stress

Mineral deficiencies are common in many women with premenstrual mood disorders. Mineral deficiencies can lead to impaired production of the brain's neurotransmitters and a weakened immune system.

Magnesium

I have used magnesium supplements extensively over more than 30 years of medical practice and have found that it is a great balancer for the nervous system. Magnesium is a mineral that is required in greater amounts in those with stress and anxiety. This is because magnesium exerts a calming effect upon the central nervous system and helps nerves and muscles to relax. When we are stressed our bodies use up far greater quantities of magnesium, and magnesium deficient people overreact to minor stress.

Magnesium can often greatly reduce many of the symptoms of stress and anxiety and will help those with the following problems:

- Depression
- Anxiety
- Panic attacks
- Period pains
- Constipation
- Muscle cramps, twitches and muscle pain
- Fibromyalgia
- Whole body tremor
- Poor sleep
- High blood pressure
- Racing heartbeat and palpitations
- Abdominal cramps and irritable bowel
- Urinary frequency
- Asthma attacks
- Migraine and tension headaches

I use a tablet called Magnesium Complete, which combines different types of magnesium salts – namely magnesium phosphate, magnesium aspartate, magnesium orotate, magnesium citrate and magnesium amino acid chelate. The dose is 1 to 2 tablets twice daily, and this provides 200 to 400 mg of pure elemental magnesium respectively. I avoid magnesium supplements containing magnesium oxide, as this form of magnesium salt is not well absorbed from the gut into the bloodstream or cells.

You can also get an Ultra Potent Magnesium Powder, which contains 4 different types of magnesium and the amino acid taurine. One teaspoon of this powder gives you 400mg of pure elemental magnesium and some women with PMS or period pains require this high dose. This powder is stirred into water or juice and is best taken one hour before retiring. Taurine is also a calming agent and relaxes the nerves and the muscles thereby improving the effect of magnesium. Supplements of magnesium and taurine can help those with premenstrual headaches and difficult to control epilepsy. Magnesium supplements can safely be taken along with anticonvulsant drugs or antidepressant drugs.

Magnesium supplements are excellent for those under stress caused by a high physical or mental workload.

The mineral magnesium, along with vitamin B 6, is required for the conversion of the amino acid tryptophan, into the happy brain chemical serotonin.

Depression associated with irritability and agitation, may be part of a magnesium deficiency syndrome. Magnesium is often called the *great relaxer* as it helps to reduce nervous and muscular tension and promotes deep restful sleep.

For more information on Magnesium, see the book titled *Magnesium - The Miracle Mineral – You won't believe the difference it makes to your health and your sex life!*

Selenium

Selenium is frequently deficient in soils in many areas of the world and foods grown in these soils contain inadequate selenium levels. A 5 week double blind crossover study, involving 50 volunteers who received a daily supplement containing either selenium or placebo found that selenium was associated with improvement in mood. The lower their initial dietary selenium intake, the more the mood improved. Selenium is also important for immune function, and severe depression can lead to an impaired immune system.

Common signs of selenium deficiency include –

- Depression
- Mental fatigue
- Reduced fertility
- Thyroid problems
- Frequent viral infections such as influenza, upper respiratory tract infections, glandular fever, swollen glands etc.
- Recurrent viral infections, such as herpes, shingles or warts
- Increased allergies and chemical sensitivities
- Recurrent warts - skin and/or genital
- Abnormal PAP smears, due to persistent human papilloma virus (HPV) in the cervix

For these problems I recommend a supplement of selenomethionine in a dose of 100 to 300mcg daily.

Tyrosine

Tyrosine is required for the manufacture of several important brain chemicals, called neurotransmitters. The production of the powerful neurotransmitters called dopamine, noradrenalin and adrenalin depends on adequate tyrosine levels in the brain. Each of these neurotransmitters helps to regulate mood and emotions.

Low dopamine levels have been linked with –

- Food cravings (particularly for carbohydrates)
- Excessive hunger and compulsive overeating
- Reduced ability to achieve satisfaction
- Reduced ability to experience pleasure
- Reduced concentration and mental drive

These symptoms become worse premenstrually when progesterone levels fall, worsening the dopamine deficiency.

Why would it be beneficial to supplement with tyrosine?

Some women have a higher requirement for tyrosine than others. Poor diet, poor appetite and poor digestion, as well as genetic factors may be responsible for this. Poor protein digestion is common in people with irritable bowel syndrome, gluten intolerance and those taking antacid medication. Chronic stress impairs digestion because it reduces the production of digestive enzymes and stomach acid. Neurotransmitters in the brain can become depleted due to stress, alcohol and sugar. Each of these factors increases the requirement for tyrosine. Some women with Premenstrual depression find tyrosine lifts their mood, concentration and mental drive. Tyrosine is an amino acid found in protein containing foods such as milk and cheese, chicken, fish, almonds, bananas and avocados.

Supplementation with pure tyrosine may provide the following benefits:

- Improved concentration, motivation and alertness
- Increased ability to experience satisfaction and pleasure
- Reduction in depression
- Reduced appetite and less tendency to binge on food
- More efficient metabolism, due to improved thyroid hormone production
- Improved energy levels

How to take tyrosine

Tyrosine is best taken away from protein foods. It can be taken with fruit or a non-dairy drink.

It can be taken two or three times daily and usually works within 15 to 20 minutes. The recommended dose is 2 grams, two or three times daily. Tyrosine can be taken in the form of a pure white powder and is tasteless and odorless. This powder can be eaten off a spoon or stirred into water or juice. Tyrosine is not addictive or habit-forming and indeed can be most helpful for those trying to quit an addiction to cigarettes, alcohol or recreational drugs.

Contraindication to tyrosine

Tyrosine supplements must not be used by people taking a type of antidepressant medication called monoamine oxidase inhibitors

(MAOIs) unless first checking with their doctor. Examples of these drugs include *Nardil* (phenelzine), *Parnate* (tranylcypromine), *Selgene* and *Eldepryl* (selegiline). Tyrosine can cause a severe rise in blood pressure in people taking these medications.

Hypericum

The herb Hypericum, also known as Saint John's wort, has been used since ancient Greek times as a remedy for nervous complaints. The clinical success of Hypericum extracts for the treatment of patients with depression has been confirmed in a large number of placebo-controlled double-blind studies. One great benefit of Hypericum is that in the doses used in humans it is usually free of side effects. Allergic reactions can occur in those who are generally allergic to herbs and may manifest as photo-sensitivity rashes when exposed to sunshine.

Hypericum is thought to exert its antidepressant and mood elevating effect in a similar way to the Mono-Amine-Oxidase Inhibitor (MAOI) antidepressant drugs. In other words it is able to inhibit the enzymes that break down the brain chemicals noradrenalin and serotonin.

Most studies demonstrating that Hypericum is an effective antidepressant have used a standardized extract of the herb which gives a dose of 900mcg total hypericin three times daily. This is equivalent to tablets containing 300mg of a 6:1 extract of the herb. One 300mg tablet, three times daily, has been found to be the generally effective therapeutic dose, although some people will find that they only need to take one or two tablets daily.

High levels of scientific and clinical evidence have shown that Hypericum is a first line treatment in the management of mild depression.

Warning – Hypericum should not be taken with certain drugs because adverse interactions may occur – these include other antidepressant drugs, blood thinners and the oral contraceptive pill. Check with your own doctor before taking Hypericum containing products.

Antidepressant Nutrients	Food Sources
Omega 3 fatty acids	Oily fish (salmon, sardines, mackerel, anchovies, tuna, trout, herrings), fish oil, krill oil, flaxseeds, walnuts, green leafy vegetables, organic eggs.
Magnesium	Green leafy vegetables, green leafy herbs, nuts, seeds, molasses, kelp
Zinc	Seafood, miso, red meat, liver, mushrooms, green leafy vegetables
Vitamin D	Sunlight, oily fish, liver, cod liver oil, milk, eggs
Vitamin B 12 (cyanocobalamin)	Meat, seafood, dairy products, organic or free-range eggs, poultry
Vitamin C	Citrus fruits, capsicum, parsley, kiwi fruit, berries, pawpaw, mango, tomato
Vitamin B 3 (niacin)	Poultry, seafood, red meat, liver, tomato, lettuce, mushrooms
Vitamin B 1 (thiamine)	Tuna, peas, eggplant, sunflower seeds, mushrooms, asparagus, spinach, celery
Vitamin B 2 (riboflavin)	Dairy products, eggs, mushroom, liver, asparagus, broccoli, spinach
Vitamin B 5 (pantothenic acid)	Eggs, yogurt, strawberries, tomato, sunflower seeds, liver, mushrooms, broccoli, cauliflower

Vitamin B 6 (pyridoxine)	Mushroom, cabbage, banana, garlic, bell peppers (capsicum), seafood, spinach, cauliflower, asparagus
Folic acid	Green leafy vegetables, cauliflower, asparagus, lentils
Potassium	Molasses, mushrooms, cucumber, squash, fennel, silverbeet, spinach, lettuce, bananas, most fruits
Tryptophan	Seafood, poultry, meat, dairy products, avocados, eggs, wheat germ, banana
Tyrosine	Milk and cheese, poultry, fish, almonds, bananas, red meat and avocados, eggs
Iodine	Seaweed, iodised salt, wild (not farmed) fish
Dopamine and noradrenalin rich foods	Avocados, lima beans, bananas, almonds, pumpkin seeds, sesame seeds, cheese

Table 2

Vitamin D – the sunshine hormone can reduce PMS

Many researchers think of Vitamin D as a hormone rather than a simple vitamin. I agree with this because Vitamin D does exert hormone like actions in the brain and skeleton. Vitamin D is made from cholesterol in the skin. When the sun's ultraviolet B (UVB) rays penetrate the exposed skin the cholesterol is turned into Vitamin D. Vitamin D is required for a healthy nervous system and a healthy immune system.

The lack of Vitamin D during the winter months may explain why premenstrual depression can become much more severe during the seasons when less sunshine is available – this type of depression is called *seasonal affective disorder*.

In women with premenstrual depression who avoid sunshine or who live in cold climates, it is important to check the blood levels of

Vitamin D; if these are found to be low, this could be exacerbating depression, anxiety, fatigue and aches and pains (fibromyalgia).

Vitamin D deficiency is a huge problem and is widespread with 60% of people being deficient. Vitamin D deficiency is often overlooked and often not tested for in those who really need it.

In addition to skin manufacture from sunlight, Vitamin D can be found in such foods as oily fish, canned fish, cod liver oil, liver, eggs, dairy products and fortified juice. It is also available in supplement form, with the current recommendation being that you take between 400 and 1000 IU of Vitamin D 3 daily. Many people, especially those who avoid the sun or those living in cold countries, need much more than this and doses of around 5000 IU daily may be needed before you can get your blood levels of Vitamin D into the higher desirable range.

Regardless of how you get it, make sure that you have an adequate amount of Vitamin D in your body. It is easy to check your body's levels of Vitamin D with a simple blood test; if your levels are below or at the lower limit of the normal range please take a Vitamin D 3 supplement and get some sunshine on your skin. Recheck your blood levels after 4 months to ensure your Vitamin D increases to the higher limit of the normal range. Make sure that you do not become deficient in Vitamin D again.

Blood levels of Vitamin D

It is vitally important to ask your doctor to check your blood level of Vitamin D. The correct blood test to measure your Vitamin D level is called 25(OH) D, also called 25-hydroxy vitamin D3.

Vitamin D can be measured in two different units of measurement and in the USA the units used are ng/mL. In Australia and Canada the units of measurement are nmol/L.

The normal ranges of Vitamin D for blood tests reported by different laboratories and countries vary significantly and you will be surprised by the large range between lower normal and upper normal – *see table 3*

Lower Limit Vitamin D	Upper Limit Vitamin D
75 nmol/L	200 nmol/L
30 ng/mL	80 ng/mL

Table 3

You don't want to be average here; you want to have levels of Vitamin D that optimize your nervous system and immune system. The optimal levels of Vitamin D are higher than the average levels.

I recommend you take enough supplements of Vitamin D 3 and/or get enough sunshine to keep your serum Vitamin D levels around 150 to 200 nmol/L or 70 to 80ng/mL. Vitamin D 3 supplements are not expensive.

Excess Vitamin D intake can cause elevated blood calcium levels; so don't overdose on it - it's not a case of the more the better. Get your blood level checked every 6 months to find the dose of Vitamin D 3 that keeps you in the optimal levels.

You would think that most people living in sunny climates produce plenty of Vitamin D but I have found that over 80% of my patients have low or suboptimal levels of Vitamin D in their blood. This is because people work long hours indoors and when outside, they cover up and use sunscreen, which blocks Vitamin D production in the skin. So if you are depressed and low in Vitamin D you should spend some time relaxing in the sun with minimal clothes on. As a guide, Dr. Craig Hassed who is senior lecturer at Monash University's Department of General Practice, recommends you need 10–15 minutes of sunshine daily if most of your skin is exposed and the UV index is 7. If the UV index is 3 and you have more clothes on you will need 25 minutes in the sun. If you are older or of dark complexion you will need more time in the sun. Avoid the midday sun in the middle of summer to prevent sunburn. It is wise to expose more skin to sunshine and take a Vitamin D supplement if your levels are low and you may find that your premenstrual syndrome reduces significantly.

10. Premenstrual Syndrome and the Thyroid Gland

A sluggish thyroid gland will not produce adequate amounts of thyroid hormone. A deficiency of thyroid hormone can affect the function of the ovaries in a very negative way. Low thyroid function often leads to problems with ovulation and subsequent lack of progesterone.

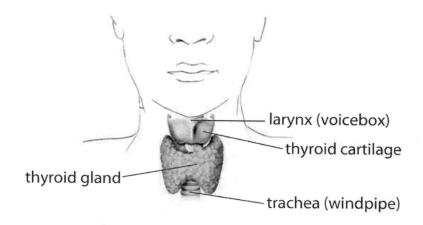

The lack of progesterone will cause some of the typical symptoms below -

- Heavy periods
- Painful periods
- Endometrial hyperplasia
- Premenstrual headaches
- Fibroids or adenomyosis of the uterus
- Endometriosis
- Unexplained infertility
- Polycystic ovarian syndrome
- Premenstrual syndrome/moodiness

- Postnatal depression
- Worsening of thyroid conditions
- Iron deficiency
- Infrequent or irregular periods
- Hair loss
- Worsening of autoimmune diseases
- Breast pain
- Breast lumpiness
- Osteoporosis
- Insomnia

As we all know, low progesterone causes PMS and especially depression and anxiety.

All women with PMS and/or menstrual problems, need a blood test to check the level of their thyroid hormones. These blood tests are very accurate. In depressed patients who also complain of fatigue, poor memory, elevated cholesterol and difficulty losing weight, it is vital to do a blood test to check the function of the thyroid gland.

The condition of low or underactive thyroid gland function is quite common. Despite this, treatment is often delayed, which is a pity as, if we optimize thyroid gland function we can get a remarkable improvement in mood and energy levels. If blood tests reveal a clearly underactive thyroid gland, it is easy to relieve the symptoms of this by giving thyroid hormone tablets or capsules. Some patients respond better by taking both types of thyroid hormone (namely Oroxine and Tertroxin) or porcine thyroid extract.

If the thyroid gland is only slightly underactive, we can often revitalize its function with supplements containing Vitamin D3, iodine, selenium and zinc. These are all contained in the correct amounts in *Thyroid Health Capsules*. (see www.liverdoctor.com)

A blood test should be done 3 months after commencing Thyroid Health Capsules to see if the thyroid function has become normal. If thyroid function has become normal, there is no need for thyroid hormone tablets; but continue to check your thyroid function with a six monthly blood test with your doctor.

If a person is low in the minerals selenium and iodine (and these deficiencies are very common), the function of their thyroid gland will be sluggish; this can cause premenstrual syndrome, fatigue, mental slowness, moodiness and unexplained infertility. *Thyroid Health Capsules™* are designed to provide adequate amounts of iodine, selenium, zinc and Vitamin D3 for optimal thyroid function. Thyroid Health Capsules do not contain hormones and do not require a prescription. *Thyroid Health Capsules™* do not contain any synthetic substances and can be taken safely with your thyroid hormone tablets. For more info call 623 334 3232 in the USA or email ehelp@liverdoctor.com

Overactive Thyroid Gland

An overactive thyroid gland can cause symptoms of anxiety – namely tremor, racing heartbeat, palpitations, diarrhea, weight loss and agitation. An overactive thyroid gland can cause the menstrual cycle to change dramatically and it may become very irregular, infrequent or much lighter or absent. An overactive thyroid gland will increase premenstrual agitation.

Once again it's important to check the thyroid gland function with a simple blood test.

Natural progesterone can help to balance both an overactive and an underactive thyroid gland.

Hormones and Body Temperature

It is interesting to note that two hormones affect the body temperature and thus the metabolism of a woman – these hormones are natural progesterone and thyroid hormone and they both increase body temperature.

After ovulation the production of progesterone by the corpus luteum gland in the ovaries increases the body temperature by 0.3 to 0.5 degrees Celsius.

A low body temperature after the expected time of ovulation, can be a sign of lack of progesterone due to absent ovulation or poor function of the corpus luteum.

A continually low body temperature can be a sign of an underactive thyroid gland.

By administering natural progesterone and improving thyroid function (with nutrients such as selenium, iodine, zinc and vitamin D) we can increase body temperature and metabolism; this is very beneficial for weight loss in many women with PMS and a sluggish thyroid gland. This will often help women with unexplained infertility.

Blood tests for thyroid function

There are many different ways to diagnose a thyroid condition. We will look at the tests your doctor or specialist can carry out, as well as tests you can do yourself at home. The earlier a thyroid problem is picked up, the better the outcome.

The blood test to check thyroid hormone levels is called a thyroid function test. This test checks levels of the following hormones:

• Thyroid Stimulating Hormone (TSH)

• Free Thyroxine (Free T4 or FT4)

• Free Triiodothyronine (Free T3 or FT3)

Free means that the hormones are not bound to carrier proteins in the blood and they are active. TSH is produced by the pituitary gland and it regulates T4 and T3 hormone production by the thyroid. If your thyroid gland cannot manufacture enough T4, TSH rises; if it produces too much T4, TSH will fall.

A thyroid function test is the main way of diagnosing thyroid disease, as well as monitoring doses of thyroid hormone medication in people with a thyroid disease. Knowing your free T3 level is important because it indicates how well your body is converting T4 into its active form T3.

The standard reference ranges for a thyroid function test used by most laboratories are:

TSH	0.30-4.50 mIU/L
Free Thyroxine (FT4)	8-22 pmol/L (or 0.7-2.0 ng/dL)
Free T3 (FT3)	2.5-6.0 pmol/L (or 260-480 pg/dL)

The reference ranges for thyroid function tests were based on statistical averages. New research is showing that the TSH reference range may not be accurate and/or desirable; the upper limit of normal TSH is ideally 2 mIU/L. The reason for this is that thyroid disease is extremely common and a large percentage of apparently healthy individuals are in the process of developing a thyroid condition.

Based on new research, the revised ideal reference range for TSH is 0.3-2.0mIU/L.

Research has shown that anyone with a TSH value above 2.0mIU/L is likely to be in the early stages of hypothyroidism!

The following statement was issued by the American National Academy of Clinical Biochemistry in their press release, issued January 18th, 2001:

"Even though a TSH level between 3.0 and 5.0 mIU/L is in the normal range, it should be considered suspect since it may signal a case of evolving thyroid underactivity."

According to the National Academy of Clinical Biochemistry, more than 95 percent of normal, healthy people have a TSH level below 2.5 mIU/L. Anyone with a higher level is likely to have underlying Hashimoto's disease or another thyroid disease which has not yet progressed to full blown hypothyroidism.

It is vital to find out as soon as possible if you have a thyroid disease, while it is still treatable with diet and nutritional intervention. If detected too late, and there is already thyroid damage, you will need to take thyroid hormone replacement for the rest of your life.

Who Should Have a Blood Test for Thyroid Disease?

Having a blood test for your thyroid gland is an important part of maintaining your health. According to the American Thyroid Association, everyone should have their thyroid gland function tested at age 35 and every five years thereafter.

If you fall into one of the categories below, you should have a complete thyroid function test (TSH, FT4 and FT3), as well as a thyroid antibody test, *at least* every five years:

- Women over the age of 35 years
- Anyone with a family history of thyroid disease or autoimmune disease
- Anyone who has previously suffered with a thyroid condition, such as postpartum thyroiditis

- Anyone with an autoimmune disease, such as type 1 diabetes, rheumatoid arthritis or lupus etc.
- People with celiac disease (gluten intolerance)
- Anyone who gains weight easily and struggles to lose it
- Anyone experiencing fatigue and lethargy
- Anyone with persistent depression
- Anyone who suffers with low fertility
- People who are taking lithium or amiodarone, as these medications are known to affect the thyroid gland
- Anyone who has received irradiation to the neck or upper chest area
- Anyone with irregular menstrual bleeding
- Anyone with very heavy menstrual bleeding

Common symptoms of hypothyroidism (underactive thyroid)

- Lethargy and fatigue
- Weight gain for no apparent reason
- Increased sensitivity to cold
- Slow heart rate (bradycardia)
- Goiter (enlarged thyroid). This will not always be present
- Dry skin and hair
- Scalp hair loss and loss of hair from the eyebrows
- Constipation
- Muscle weakness, especially of the arms and legs
- Slow reflexes
- Infertility
- Fluid retention
- Puffiness around the eyes
- Mental depression and slowness
- Irregular and/or heavy menstrual bleeding

The Temperature Test

More than 50 years ago, a doctor named Broda Barnes found that the basal (resting) body temperature is a good indicator of thyroid function. An underactive thyroid gland can produce a drop in body temperature, whereas an overactive thyroid can increase body temperature. Measuring your body temperature is another tool you can use to diagnose a problem with your thyroid gland. It should be used in conjunction with a blood test and your symptoms.

Instructions for performing the thyroid temperature test

1) It is preferable to use a mercury thermometer. Clean the thermometer with cool, soapy water. Gripping the end opposite the bulb, shake the thermometer down until it reaches 96 degrees Fahrenheit (35 degrees Celsius) or lower. Place the thermometer beside your bed within easy reach, so that you can pick it up while still lying down the next morning.

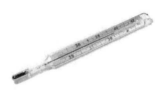

Mercury Thermometer

2) The next morning, as soon as you wake up, place the thermometer in your armpit, so that the bulb is in your armpit. Make sure that there is no clothing between your armpit and the thermometer. Hold the thermometer there for ten minutes and continue lying still. When measuring your body temperature as a test for thyroid function, it is better to place the thermometer in the armpit. When measuring your body temperature as a test for ovulation, either the armpit or under the tongue are suitable sites to place the thermometer.

3) Write down your temperature. You must do this for four consecutive days.

Important tips

Your temperature must be taken as soon as you wake up in the morning; before you have moved out of bed, eaten or had anything to drink. This way you will be recording your lowest temperature of the day. Menstruating women must perform this test starting on the second day of their period; this is because ovulation produces a rise in body temperature and would not give a true reading. Post menopausal women, and men can perform this test at any time. Do not do this test when you have an infection, injury or any other condition that can produce a mild fever.

A normal axillary (armpit) body temperature for adults is between 97.8 to 98.2 degrees Fahrenheit and 36.5 and 36.7 degrees Celsius. If your body temperature consistently falls below 97.8 degrees Fahrenheit or below (36.5 degrees Celsius), you should see your doctor for tests of your thyroid function. This method is not always 100 percent accurate and should not be relied upon solely; it can be helpful when used in conjunction with other thyroid tests.

Normal Variations of Body Temperature

Your body temperature can vary significantly depending upon which part of the body you place the thermometer to measure it.

Internal measurements (when you place the thermometer inside a body cavity such as the rectum or vagina). This is called the core body temperature. The conventionally accepted average is 37.0 °C (98.6 °F).

Oral measurements (when you place the thermometer under the tongue).

The typical oral measurement is (36.8±0.7 °C), or 98.24±1.26 °F.

Skin measurements (when you place the thermometer in the armpit (axilla))

The commonly quoted value is 36.6 °C (97.9 °F), with a range of 36.25 °C (97.25 °F) to 37.5 °C (99.5 °F)

Most people think of these numbers as representing the normal temperature; however a wide range of temperatures has been found in healthy people. In samples of adult women and men, the normal range for oral temperature is 33.2–38.2 °C (92–101 °F), for rectal temperature it is 34.4–37.8 °C (94–100 °F), and for axillary (armpit) temperature it is 35.5–37.0 °C (96–99 °F). Thus we look for trends or changes to detect changes in your metabolism and hormones. A continually decreasing temperature trend could mean your thyroid is gradually becoming under active or sluggish.

Your body temperature can be affected by -

• Time of day - the core body temperature of an individual tends to have the lowest value in the second half of the sleep cycle; this low point is called the nadir and is one of the primary markers for circadian rhythms.

• The body temperature also changes, usually decreasing, when an individual is hungry, sleepy, or cold.

• If your body weight is very low, (as in anorexia nervosa), your body temperature can be abnormally low and this conserves precious energy reserves

• If you are significantly overweight, and especially if you have a fatty liver, your core body temperature tends to be higher than if you were at a healthy weight. This can be quite uncomfortable for those people and they feel much cooler when they improve their liver function and lose weight.

The function of the ovaries and the thyroid gland are closely related

Abnormal thyroid function can cause abnormal function of the ovaries, which in turn worsens the function of the thyroid gland. In other words, it becomes a vicious circle.

We need to treat both the thyroid gland and the ovaries to restore hormonal balance. Natural progesterone is essential in such cases.

• For more in depth information on the holistic treatment of thyroid problems, see my book *Your Thyroid Problems Solved* or visit www.aboutthyroid.com or call my Women's Health Advisory Service on 623 334 3232 in the USA or 02 4655 8855 in Australia.

Farewell Message

Millions of women suffer from hormonal imbalances, from women traumatized by premenstrual syndrome, to acne, low thyroid and mothers struggling with postnatal depression or heavy menstrual bleeding. Hormonal upheavals, especially progesterone deficiency, can often be blamed for recurring headaches, sexual dysfunction, problems after hysterectomy and tubal ligation, unwanted body and/or facial hair, balding, chronic fatigue and general poor health.

The majority of women have coped admirably with such hormonal problems but, in a significant minority, these problems have had ruinous effects resulting in severe depression, family disruption, child battering, loss of self-esteem, drug addiction and even suicide. It can be very frightening to feel a victim of one's hormones, knowing that month after month unpleasant symptoms will recur to remind us of our uniquely female vulnerability.

When we understand that the hormonal system of a woman is such a delicate and complex network of interacting body chemicals, it is not surprising that, at times, it seems to go haywire! Not only are we vulnerable to our hormonal fluctuations but our hormones are influenced by our weight, lifestyle, exercise patterns, environmental chemicals, stress, diet, nutritional imbalances and increasing age.

To fine tune our hormones is obviously a very specialized and complicated endeavour. It is now possible for the first time in history to achieve this because of new breakthroughs in the speciality of women's hormones (Gynecological Endocrinology).

Thankfully the attitude of society and doctors towards women with hormonal problems is changing. These problems have their hilarious side as depicted by the cartoons in this book and they also have their tragic side with a propensity to devastate the lives of many women. Doctors are finally realizing that women with hormonal problems want to be taken seriously and offered real and lasting solutions. They don't want to be stereotyped, patronized, trivialised or kept in the dark. It does not help to be told that your symptoms are inevitable, a natural part of womanhood or just a sign of your age.

I have written this book because I am continually challenged with women, whose lives are being turned upside down by their hormones. These women are not neurotic or inadequate. They are intelligent, articulate, strong and very relatable personalities. They recognize that powerful hormonal imbalances are causing mental and/or physical changes that they need help to control so that their lives can be productive, fulfilled and stable.

I, myself, have had to find solutions for my own hormonally caused health problems that were preventing me from enjoying my life and 'getting on with it', so to speak. Thus I know how it feels to be a victim of one's hormones and thankfully, I now know how to gain control over my own hormonal demons. To have overcome these horrible symptoms in myself and thousands of my patients, has given me great satisfaction, confidence and compassion.

I hope that this book enables me to share with you my many years of accumulated clinical research and experience. This book aims to give you more insight and to show you all your treatment options with an emphasis on natural hormone and nutritional therapies. It is designed to give you all the tools that you will need to work with your doctor in conquering the many hormonal problems that may befall you.

Don't forget you can email us if you need more help. ehelp@ liverdoctor.com

References

1. Abraham G.E. et al, Hormonal and behavioural changes during the menstrual cycle, Senologia. 1978: 3:33

2. Backstrom CT, et al, Persistence of symptoms of PMT in hysterectomised women, British Journal Obstets & Gynaec. 1981: 88:530

3. Dr Katharina Dalton's original Books (limited availability via amazon.com)
   Once a Month - Understanding & Treating PMS, Published by Hunter House
   PMS: The Essential Guide to Treatment Options, Hunter House publishers CA, USA
   Depression After Childbirth
   PMS and Progesterone therapy, Published by Year Book Medical Pub

4. Dalton K, 1970, Brit Med Journ., 2:27

5. Dalton K, 1976, Proceedings Royal Society of Medicine, 59:10, 1014

6. Watson, NR, et al, Gynaec Endocrinol. 4:99-107, 1990

7. Bavernfeind, JC, Vit B6: nutritional & pharmaceutical usage, Pg 78-110, Nat Acad of Sciences, Washington 1978

8. Abraham G, et al, RBC Magnesium in premenopausal women, International Clinical Nutrition Review, Vol 3, No 1, 1983

9. American Journal of Obstetrics & Gynecology. June 1999, 180(6): 1504-11

10. The PEPI Trial; The Post Menopausal Estrogen Progestin Interventions Trial, Effects of HRT on endometrial histology in postmenopausal women, JAMA, 1996, February; 275(5):370-375 and November 276 (17):1430-32 and JAMA 1997, May; 277(19):1515

11. The WHI Study, The Risks & Benefits of Estrogen & Progestin in healthy post-menopausal women, JAMA, Vol 288, No.3, July 17th 2002

12. The Journal of the Climacteric and Postmenopause, Maturitas 20 (1995) 191-198

13. Kent Holtorf, MD - Postgraduate Medicine, Volume 121, Issue 1, January 2009 - https://www.sandracabot.com/bioidentical-hormone-debate

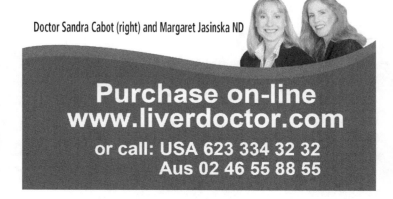

Infertility:
the hidden causes

**In this well researched book, Dr Sandra Cabot and
naturopath Margaret Jasinska explore the many hidden
causes of infertility which are often easily overcome.**

*One in six couples experience infertility. They are often left confused,
hopeless and with no definitive answers as to what can be done
to improve their chance of conceiving. Infertility is not a disease;
rather it is a symptom of an underlying health problem.*

*By improving the health of both prospective parents, not only will this
dramatically increase the chance of achieving a healthy pregnancy;
it will also increase the likelihood of having a healthy baby.*

In this book Dr Sandra Cabot and naturopath Margaret Jasinska help you to
overcome problems that compromise fertility, such as:

- Endometriosis
- Balance your hormones naturally
- Overcome polycystic ovarian syndrome
- Overcome immune system disorders
- Reduce exposure to environmental chemicals
- Overcome hidden infections
- Vitamin and/or mineral deficiencies
- Understand tests you must have when trying to conceive

- Identify and overcome factors that lead to male infertility
- Increase sperm counts and improve the quality of sperm
- Improve your chance of success with IVF
- Maintain a healthy pregnancy
- Reduce the risk of miscarriage
- Give your baby the best possible start in life

This is what you will find at:

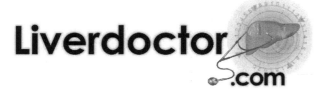

Liverdoctor.com

Holistic medical information

Well researched and up-to-date information to help you in your daily life
Informative on-line information to assist you look after your health and weight

Free liver check up test

Take this liver check up and receive private & confidential feedback on
the state of your liver and general health - www.liverdoctor.com/liver-check

Health supplements

Including Doctor Cabot's Livatone Plus capsules to support optimal liver function

On-line shopping

Sandra Cabot MD has a excellent range of health products and publications

On-line help from Dr Cabot's Team

Confidential and expert help from Dr Cabot's highly trained nutritionists and
naturopaths. Simply email us at ehelp@liverdoctor.com

Free LIVERISH newsletter

Register on-line for the free LIVERISH nesletter at www.liverdoctor.com/newsletter

Love you liver and live longer

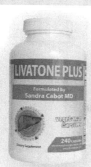
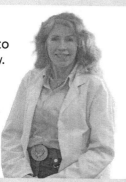
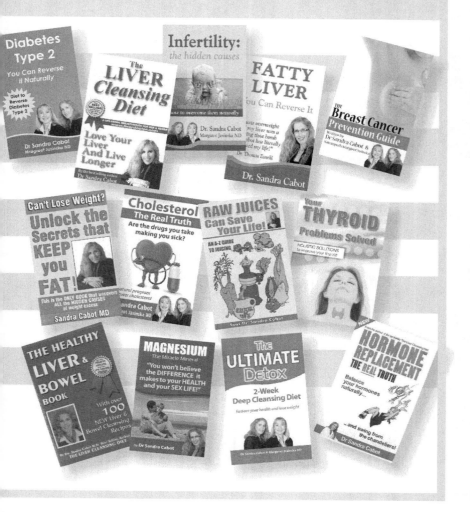